COLOR ATLAS OF THE DISEASES OF FISHES, AMPHIBIANS AND REPTILES

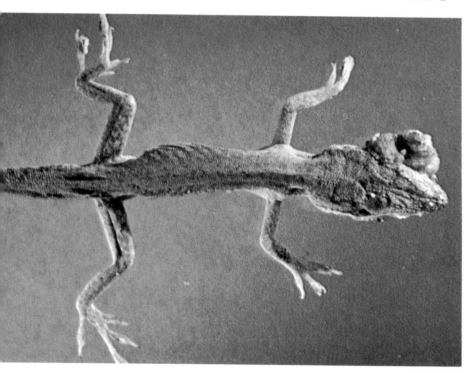

E. ELKAN, M.D.
Department of Histopathology
Mt. Vernon Hospital
Northwood, Middlesex, U.K.
and
H.-H. REICHENBACH-KLINKE, PH.D.
Professor for Zoology and Fisheries
University of Munich, Germany

in collaboration with Marsha Landolt

ISBN 0-87666-028-6

Distributed in the U.S.A. by T.F.H. Publications, Inc., 211 West Sylvania Avenue, P.O. Box 27, Neptune City, N.J. 07753; in England by T.F.H. (Gt. Britain) Ltd., 13 Nutley Lane, Reigate, Surrey; in Canada to the book store and library trade by Clarke, Irwin & Company, Clarwin House, 791 St. Clair Avenue West, Toronto 10, Ontario; in Canada to the pet trade by Rolf C. Hagen Ltd., 3225 Sartelon Street, Montreal 382, Quebec; in Southeast Asia by Y.W. Ong, 9 Lorong 36 Geylang, Singapore 14; in Australia and the south Pacific by Pet Imports Pty. Ltd., P.O. Box 149, Brookvale 2100, N.S.W., Australia. Published by T.F.H. Publications Inc., Ltd., The British Crown Colony of Hong Kong.

CONTENTS

Acknowledgments

The authors wish to express their sincere gratitude to the contributors mentioned below, who have allowed examples of their work to be included.

Equally they are much obliged to Marsha Landolt for her devotion in adjusting and editing the material contributed by the authors.

Crewehr: page 176

Dr. W. Foersch: page 43, top

Henschel: page 127

Kipp, Munich: page 69

Korting: page 147, top

Dr. Krampitz, Munich: pages 95, bottom; 96, top

Negele, Munich: page 90.

Dr. H.-H. Reichenbach-Klinke: pages 56, top; 77, top; 91, top; 120, bottom; 139; 144, bottom; 147, bottom; 152, top; 153; 170; 196, bottom; 214; 215; 216; 246

Dr. S.F. Snieszko: 26, top

Zool. -Par. Inst., Munich: 11, bottom; 15, bottom; 53, top; 101, bottom; 125; 143; 145; 159; 166, top; 174; 186; 212; 217; 218, bottom.

Preface

When we published the *Principal Diseases of Lower Vertebrates* in 1965, it was economically impossible to include all the illustrations in color which were, even at that time, available to us. In the intervening years our collection of color slides has grown, and we are most gratified that T.F.H. Publications, Inc., publisher of the three volume American edition of *Principal Diseases,* has decided to bear the expense of publishing this companion to our first volumes in the form of an atlas showing most of our pictures in color.

Obviously, even including this latest attempt, we cannot hope to present a complete text of lower vertebrate pathology. The worker in this field depends on the material available to him, may it come from his own collection or from friends and institutions overseas. This material, however, even if collected unsystematically, is in many instances of great interest, and if its publication serves no other purpose, it may at least form the basis of a complete text of lower vertebrate pathology which will certainly be written in the foreseeable future.

Daily experience has shown that the amateur is not very interested in scientific minutiae, but that what he wants to know, and in the simplest terms, is an answer to the question: why did this animal die? A large choice of illustrations taken from typical cases may help him to find, if not the complete answer, a close approximation to it. If readers in distant, especially tropical countries should look in vain for conditions occurring in their own area, they might consider the difficulties of material from such region reaching an institute where it can be properly investigated. As far as virology and bacteriology are concerned, both of which play an important role, a useful diagnosis can only be made on the spot. In the other categories of causes of death the requirements are not quite so stringent, but it cannot be repeated too often that material should reach the laboratory alive or at least well preserved. Neglect at this first stage often makes further investigation either unnecessarily difficult or impossible.

When comparing any of the pictures in this *Atlas* with material of his own, the reader should not be discouraged by slight color discrepancies. No two cases, even of the same disease, ever look exactly alike at autopsy, and microscopic sections are presented in colors of the technician's choice, which may vary from case to case. Even considering the limits of color reproduction, the advantage of a color plate over a black and white print is enormous. For us every object presents itself colored in some way, and the poor black and white illustrations which fill our textbooks and journals are, in most instances, useless. There can hardly be a scientist in the world who would not look forward to the time when the money spent on the glossy advertising pages will be spread over the whole book or journal so that every picture presents itself in its true colors.

The material available divides itself naturally into the arrangement adopted in our original text, fish, amphibia and reptiles, but it cannot follow the textbooks of human pathology and medicine which start with signs and symptoms and end with therapeutics. Unfortunately, many of the lower vertebrates show no signs and symptoms at all before they are suddenly and unexpectedly found dead and, equally unfortunately, our therapeutic armament for their diseases is still deplorably limited.

The human body may be able to withstand the innumerable medicines we prescribe, but a small fish or a little lizard may easily die before we have managed to make an impression on the bacteria or protozoa which have assailed it. What we need for these animals are drugs which selectively kill viruses, bacteria and protozoa while doing no harm to the hosts, a desideratum which at present is only a dream. Even so, common species must be kept in the best possible conditions in the places where they are used as test animals, and rare species must be looked after in the best possible way to prevent their extinction. To do this common diseases must be recognized, and of course recognition is necessary if specific treatments are ever to be developed.

We shall be satisfied if this *Atlas* helps in even a small way to achieve this goal.

E. Elkan
H. Reichenbach-Klinke

I. VIRAL DISEASES

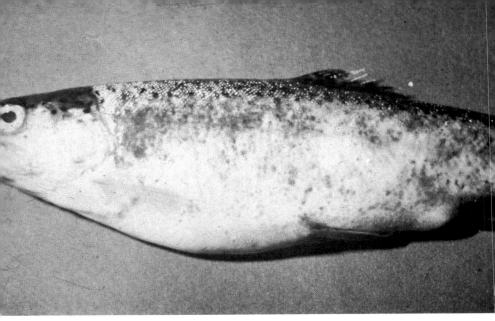

1. A rainbow trout *(Salmo gairdneri)* with dermal inflammation caused by viral hemorrhagic septicemia (VHS). The etiologic agent of this disease is a rhabdovirus. Photo: Dr. Ghittino.

2. Chronic renal form of VHS in a rainbow trout *(Salmo gairdneri)*. Photo: Dr. P. de Kinkelin.

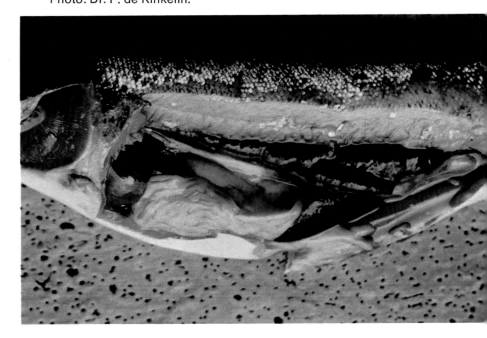

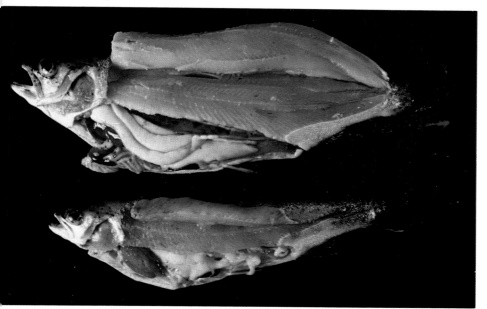

3. VHS in rainbow trout (*Salmo gairdneri*). The upper specimen is also infested with the gill parasite *Ergasilus*. Photo: Dr. Ghittino.

4. Opened rainbow trout showing typical petechial hemorrhages in the liver and musculature due to VHS. This is a severe disease with high mortality. Photo: Dr. Ghittino.

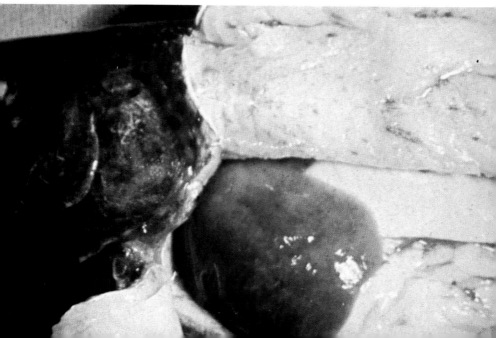

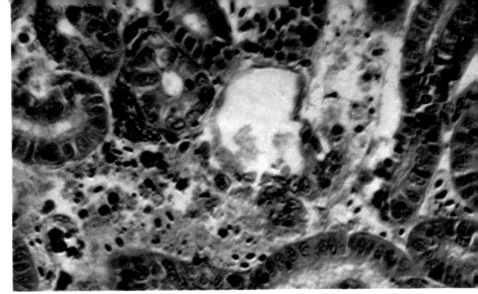

5. The kidneys of a salmonid fish affected with Infectious Hema-
topoietic Necrosis (IHN). IHN, like VHS, is caused by a rhabdovirus.
It leads to massive destruction of the blood-forming tissues.
Photo: Yasutake.

6. Infectious dropsy in a carp *(Cyprinus carpio),* chronic form with
dermal ulceration. Infectious dropsy (ID) has a high mortality rate. In
the acute form the signs are dermal inflammation, exophthalmos,
ascites and hemorrhage of the swimbladder and the muscles. Like
VHS and IHN, the etiologic agent is a rhabdovirus. Superinfection
with aeromonad bacteria often occurs.

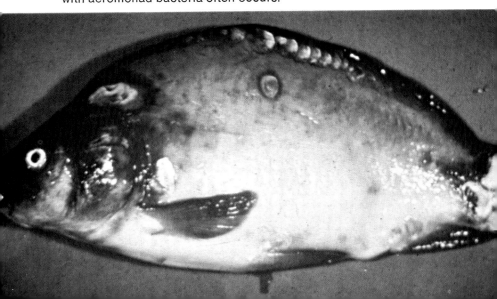

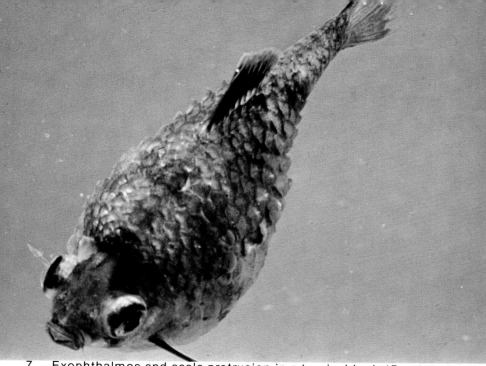

7. Exophthalmos and scale protrusion in a tropical barb (Cyprinidae). These are typical signs of infectious dropsy. Photo: Frickhinger.

8. Swim Bladder Inflammation (SBI) of a carp (*Cyprinus carpio*). Note the hemorrhagic condition of the swim bladder. The causative agent is a rhabdovirus. Photo: Zool. -Par. Inst. Munich.

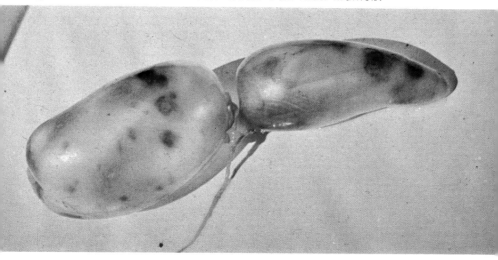

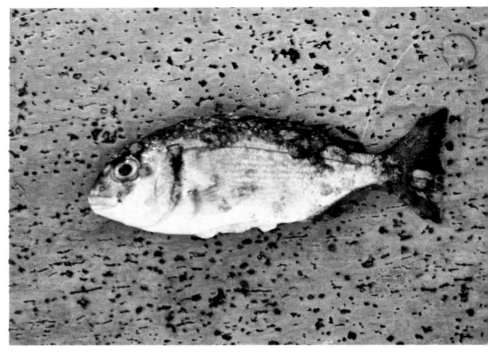

9. Lymphocystis disease of a gilthead *(Chrysophrys aurata)*. This disease is caused by an iridovirus. Photo: Dr. P. de Kinkelin.

10. Lymphocystis disease of plaice *(Pleuronectes platessa)*.

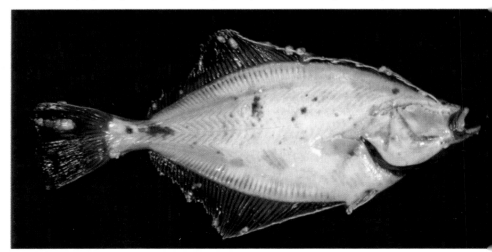

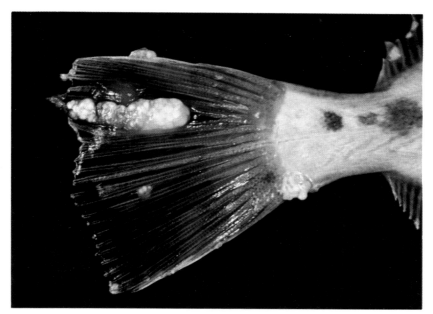

11. Lymphocystis disease of plaice *(Pleuronectes platessa)* at higher magnification.

12. Lymphocystis disease of a flounder.

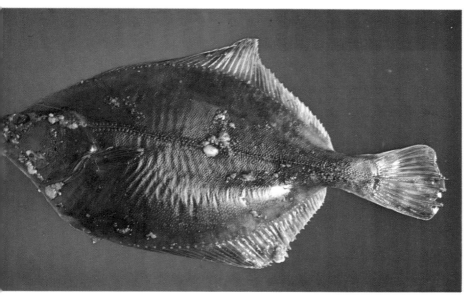

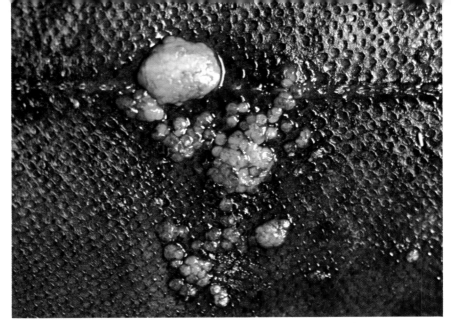

13. Lymphocystis disease of flounder at higher magnification.

14. Skin of flounder with lymphocystis disease. Note the hypertrophic epithelial cells.

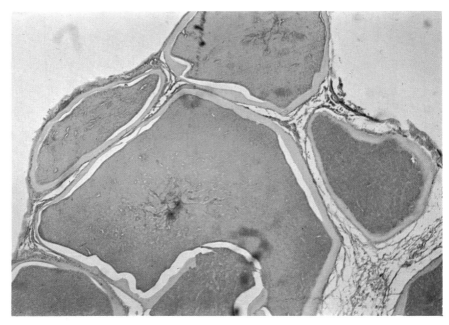

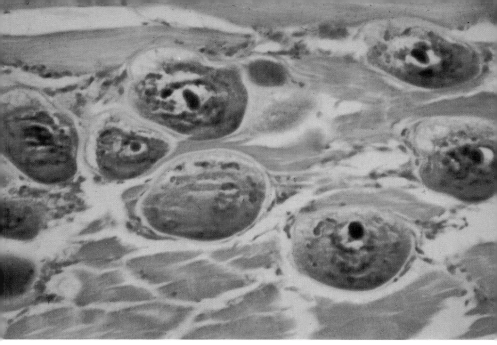

15. Skin of bluegill *(Lepomis macrochirus)* showing hypertrophied cells due to lymphocystis disease. Photo: Frickhinger.

16. Epithelioma (cauliflower disease) on the head of an eel *(Anguilla anguilla)*. While the disease is virus associated, it has not yet been proved to be caused by a virus.

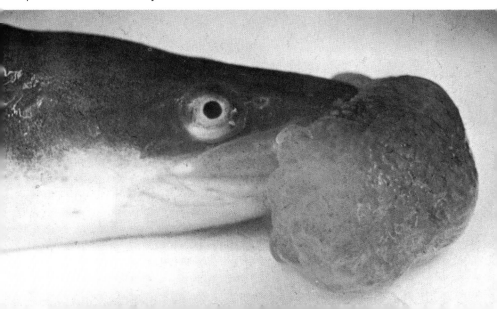

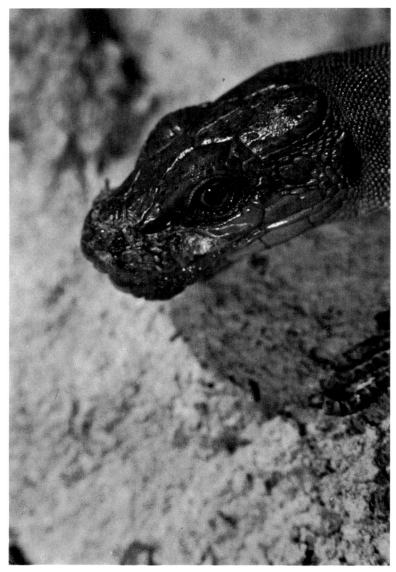

17. Dermal papillomatosis in *Lacerta sicula*. It is now well accepted that the benign papillomatous degeneration of the skin commonly known as warts is due to a viral infection. Photo: Elkan.

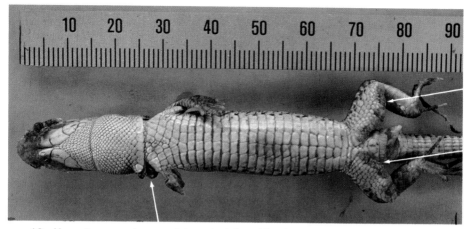

18. If warts occur in a moist part of the skin, they are often transmitted to the adjoining area. In this case the degeneration started at the lips, spread to part of the head and then to other parts of the body. Photo: Elkan.

19. This photo shows the thick layers of keratin produced by the hyperplastic skin which is thrown into long pointed folds (acanthosis). In the skin of the normal lizard no dermal papillae occur. Photo: Elkan.

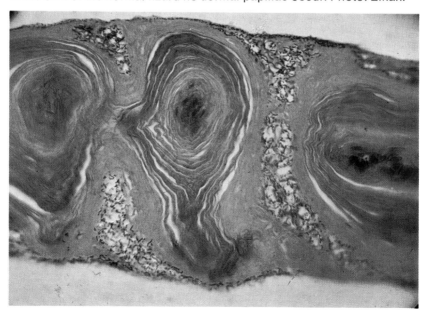

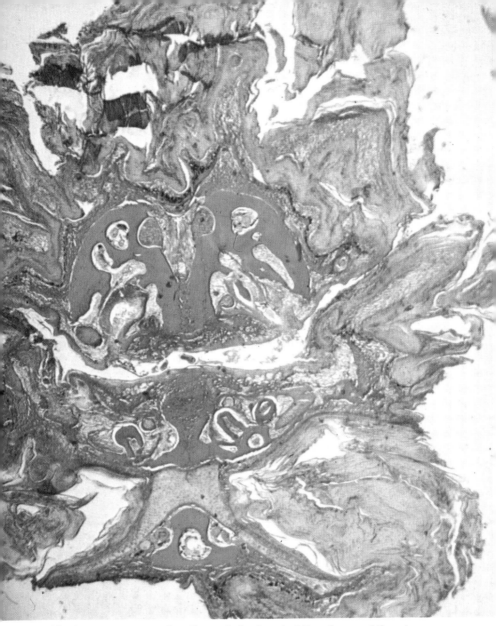

20. A transverse section through the head of the diseased lizard. Both nostrils were obstructed. The mouth, because of the masses of keratin obstructing it, could no longer be closed. Pure cultures of a saprophytic *Streptococcus* grew in the dermis and between the layers of keratin. Photo: Elkan.

II. BACTERIAL DISEASES

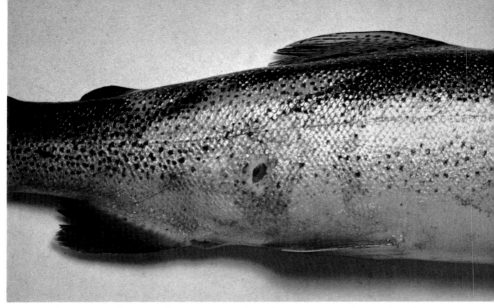

21. Furunculosis, a disease caused by *Aeromonas salmonicida,* in rainbow trout *(Salmo gairdneri).*

22. Stained smear of furuncle material to show the Gram negative bacteria.

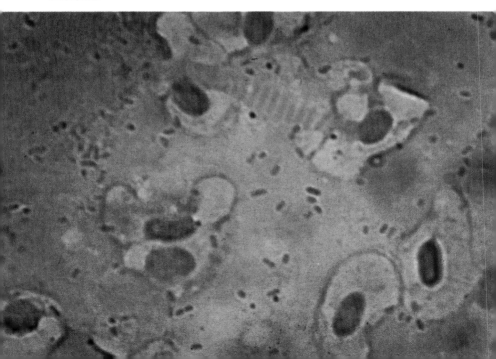

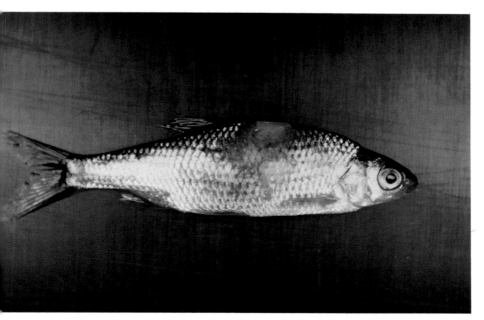

23. Hemorrhagic septicemia caused by *Aeromonas liquefaciens* in a roach *(Rutilus rutilus)*.

24. *Aeromonas liquefaciens* infection of a salmonid fish.

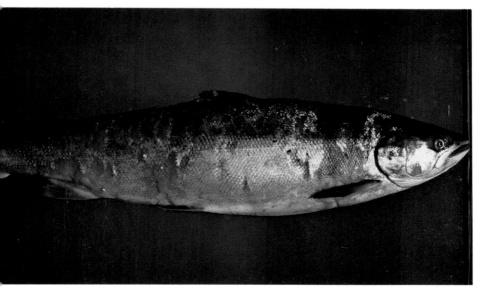

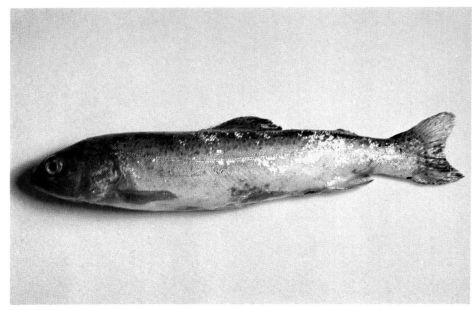

25. Hemorrhagic septicemia due to *Aeromonas liquefaciens* in a rainbow trout *(Salmo gairdneri)*.

26. Rainbow trout *(Salmo gairdneri)* with secondary *Aeromonas* infection following a heron bite.

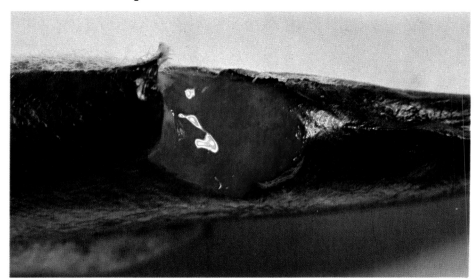

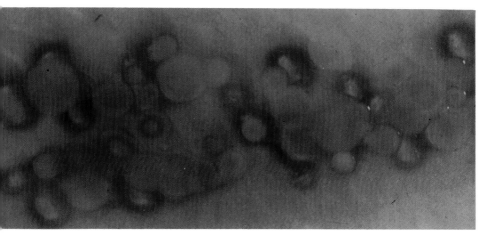

27. Colonies of *Aeromonas* sp. grown in culture.

28. One of the most serious killers of aquatic animals, particularly frogs, is *Pseudomonas,* a slender Gram negative rod which produces a toxin similar to that of diphtheria. *P. aerogenes* and *P. hydrophilus* are most commonly cited as organisms capable of wiping out a whole collection of fish or frogs within a few hours. In frogs they cause the condition commonly known as red leg, and the animals die from loss of fluid, general sepsis and septic pneumonia. The photograph shows an infected *Xenopus laevis.* Photo: Elkan.

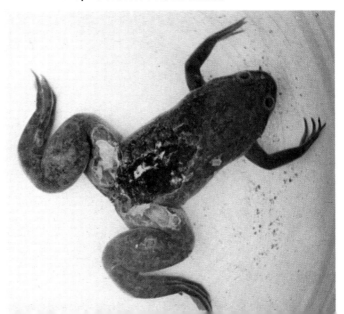

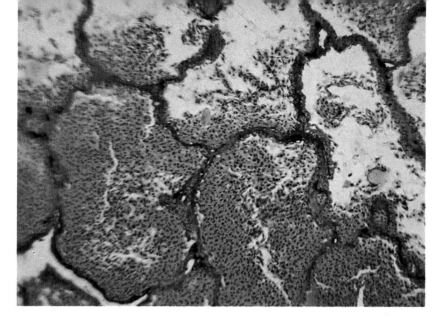

29. *Xenopus laevis* with hemorrhagic septic pneumonia caused by *Pseudomonas* sp. Photo: Elkan.

30. Saltwater rainbow trout with an external lesion accompanied by *Vibrio* sp.

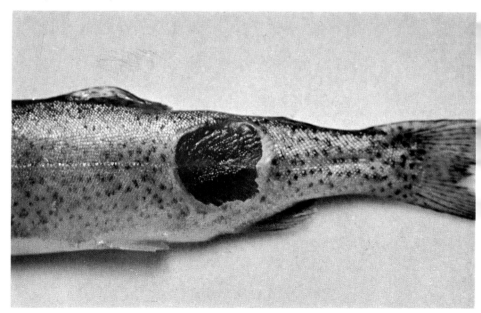

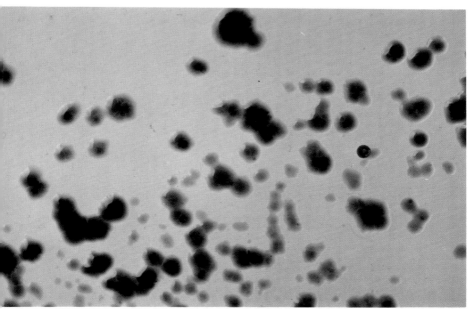

31. Colonies of *Vibrio anguillarum* grown in culture.

32. *Vibrio anguillarum* taken from the liver of a plaice *(Pleuronectes platessa). Vibrio* is a Gram negative, slightly curved rod.

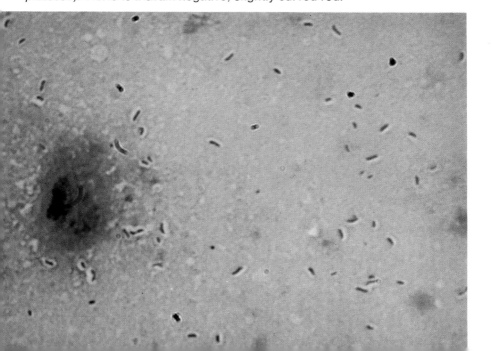

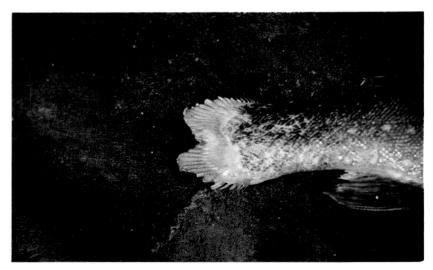

33.   Peduncle disease, or coldwater disease, is caused by the myxobacterium *Cytophaga psychrophila* and is manifested by severe erosion of the caudal region.

34.   Columnaris disease is caused by the myxobacterium *Chondrococcus columnaris*. Sometimes the soft fin tissue becomes eroded and shows necrotic gaps.

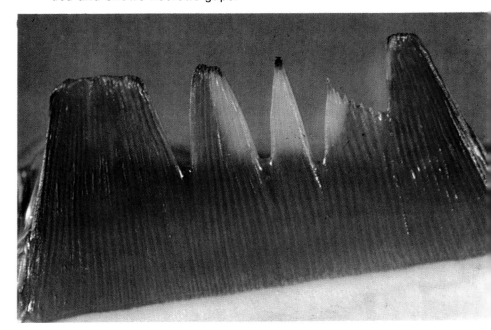

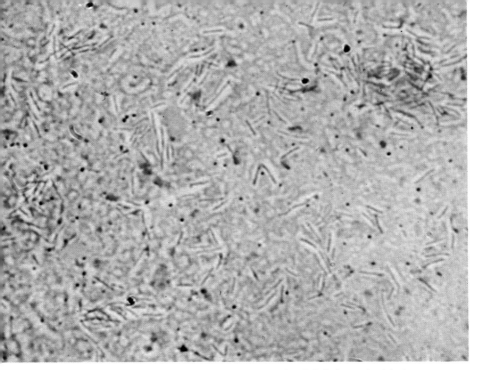

35. Gram stained smear taken from the skin of a fish infected with the myxobacterium *Chondrococcus columnaris,* a thin Gram negative rod.

36. Severe fin and tail rot in cichlids. This condition can be caused by a variety of bacteria.

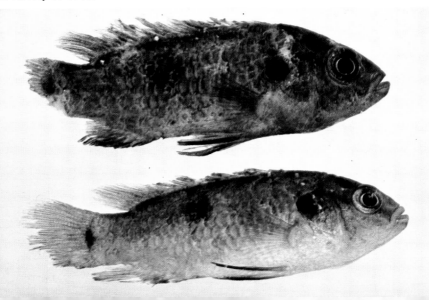

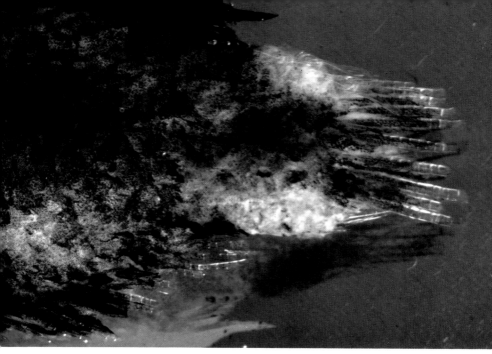

37. Bacterial tail rot in a cichlid.

38. Gram positive diplobacilli seen in a smear taken from the skin of a salmonid fish with bacterial kidney disease (KD).

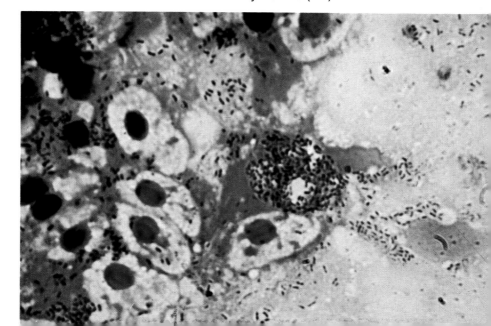

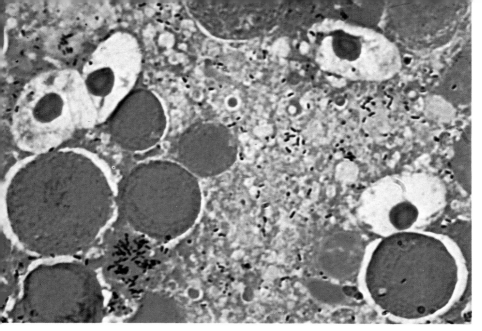

39. Gram positive diplobacilli seen in a smear taken from the kidney of a salmonid fish with KD.

40. Gram positive diplobacilli seen in a smear taken from the spleen of a salmonid fish with KD.

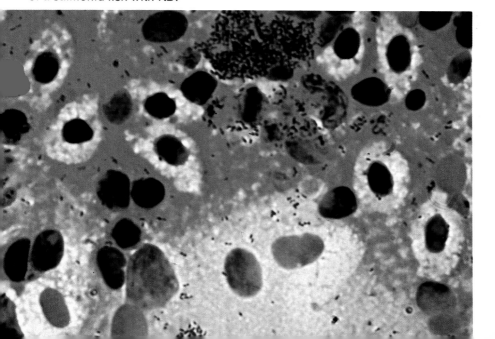

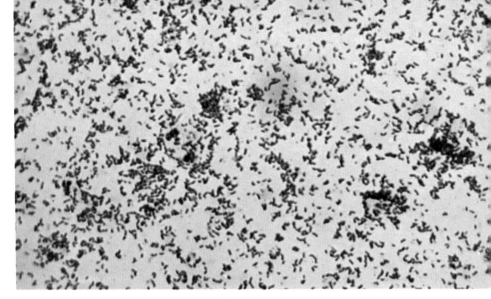

41. Kidney disease organisms (*Corynebacterium* sp.) taken from a bacterial culture.

42. Spinal curvature seen in guppies *(Poecilia reticulata)* affected with tuberculosis (TB).

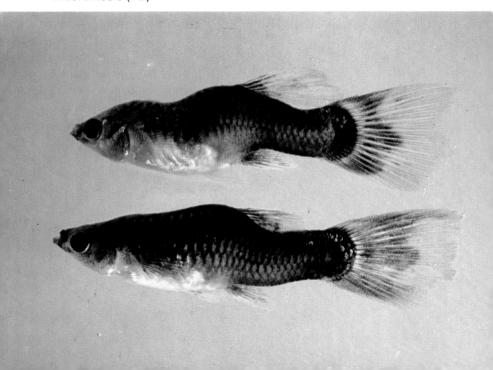

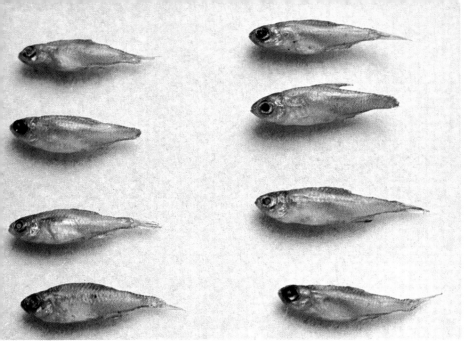

43. Fin necrosis and loss of pigmentation seen in neon tetras *(Paracheirodon innesi)* afflicted with TB.

44. Tubercles in a neon tetra *(Paracheirodon innesi)* afflicted with TB. Photo: Frickhinger.

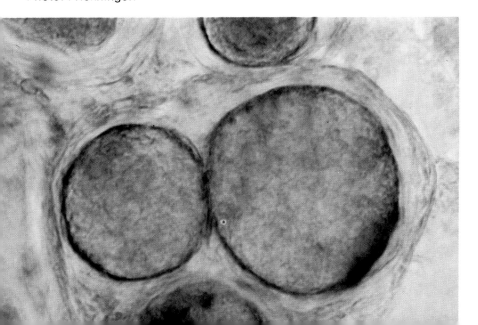

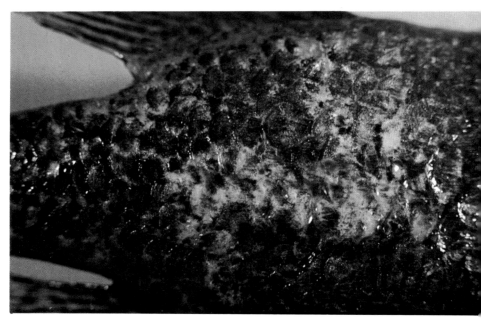

45. Skin lesion of rock bass *(Amboplites)* that has TB.

46. Tuberculosis is caused by the genus *Mycobacterium.* This photograph shows the acid fast organisms in the kidney of a coho salmon *(Oncorhynchus kisutch).*

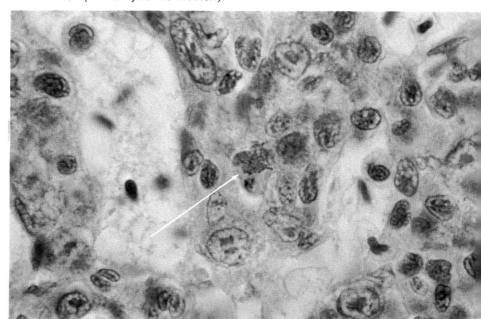

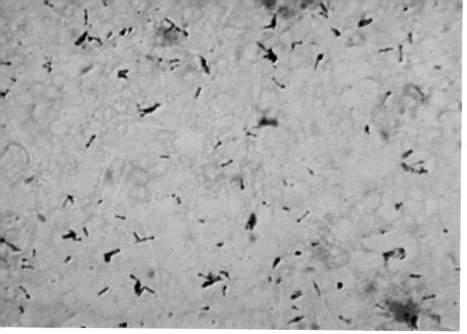

47. Acid fast *Mycobacterium* seen in a smear taken from the skin of a tropical fish with TB. Photo: Piscisan Ltd.

48. *Mycobacterium* seen in a smear taken from the kidney of a tropical fish with TB. Photo: Piscisan Ltd.

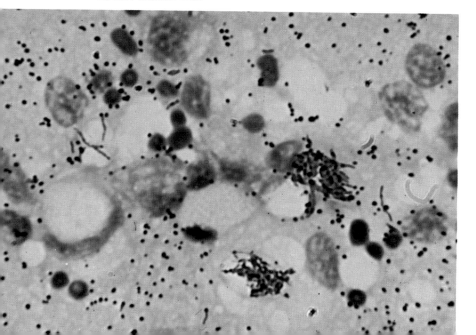

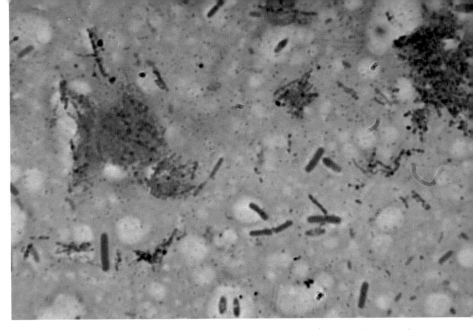

49. Acid fast *Mycobacterium* and non-acid fast bacteria seen in a smear taken from the skin of a dead tropical fish with TB. Photo: Piscisan Ltd.

50. Occasionally one sees a case of generalized tuberculous dermatitis. The ulceration gradually dissolves the layers of skin until the subcutaneous lymph sac is reached. The animals die not so much from sepsis as from loss of fluid. Photo: Elkan.

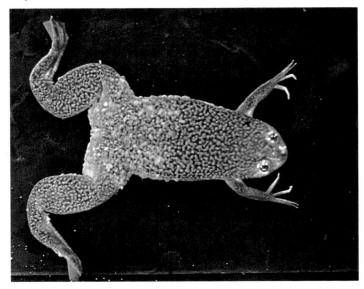

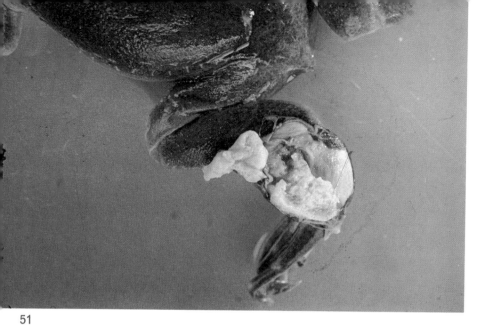

51

51-54. Photographs 51-54 show various stages in the development of
tubercles and tubercular ulceration in the leg of *Xenopus laevis*.
Photos: Elkan.

52

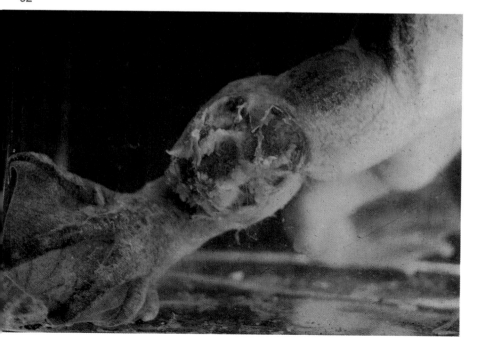

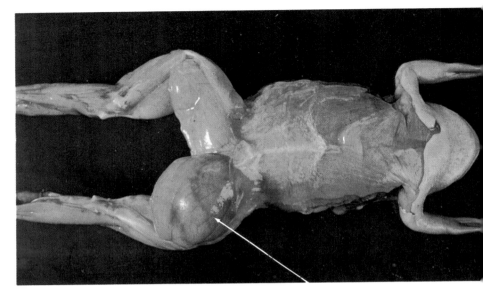

53

54

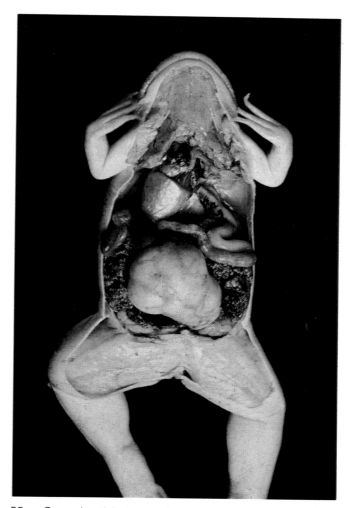

55. Grossly, this lesion is indistinguishable from carcinoma. The condition causes complete intestinal obstruction which eventually leads to the death of the frog. Rarely, even the heart may be affected by this tuberculous process. This photograph shows involvement of the large intestine. Photo: Elkan.

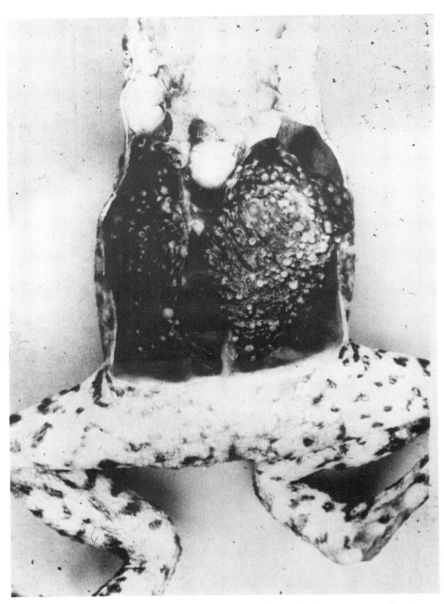

56. Once the bacteria have become disseminated, they may manifest their presence anywhere. The organ system least commonly affected is the central nervous system, while both liver and kidney usually count among the earliest sites of the tuberculous process. Photo: Elkan.

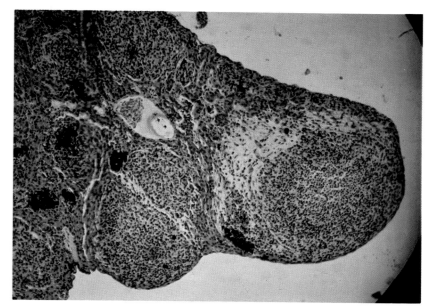

57-58. Photographs 57-58 are microscopic sections showing tubercles in livers of *Bufo bufo.* Figure 58 is selectively stained for the presence of tubercle bacilli (Ziehl-Neelsen's Carbol-Fuchsin). Photos: Elkan.

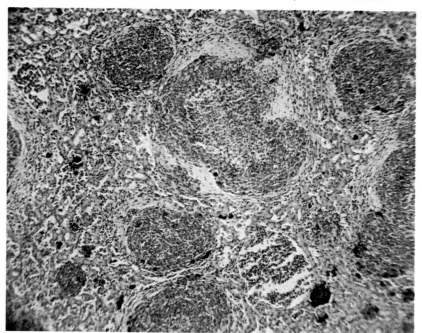

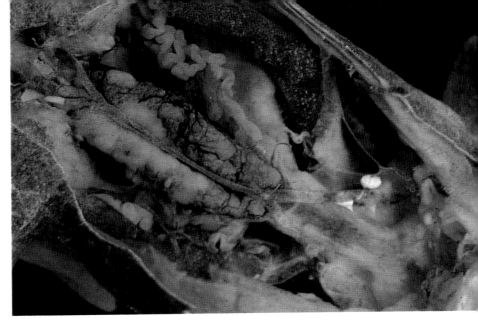

59. The kidney of *Xenopus laevis* affected by tuberculosis. It should be emphasized that it is impossible, by naked eye inspection alone, to distinguish tuberculosis of the kidney from malignant neoplastic disease. Photo: Elkan.

60. An early tubercle developing in the kidney of *Bufo bufo*. Note that in spite of the small lesion, some of the adjoining tubules are already obstructed and filled with hyaline material. Photo: Elkan.

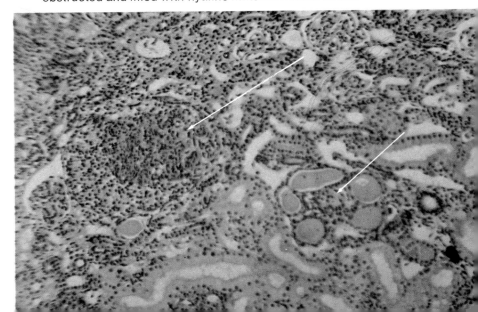

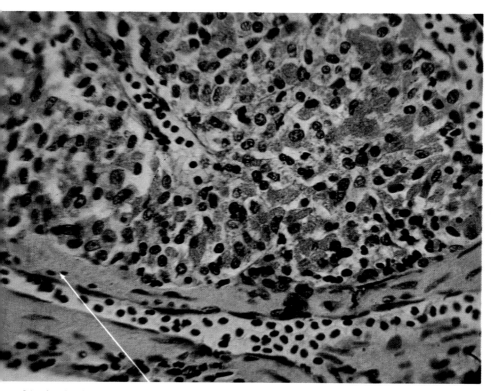

61. In the lungs, the tubercular process can produce a bizarre picture. In the case shown, the whole of the left lung was transformed into a large sausage-shaped tubercular mass, and in the right lung the same process was just starting at the base. No other organ was affected, and the pleuroperitoneum was uninvolved. The bacteria which completely destroyed the lung (upper half of frame) were unable to breach the serosal surface and break through into the body cavity. This demonstrates the low virulence of the cold-water mycobacteria which one would be inclined to place midway between saprophytes and pathogens. The arrow indicates the pleura. Photo: Elkan.

41

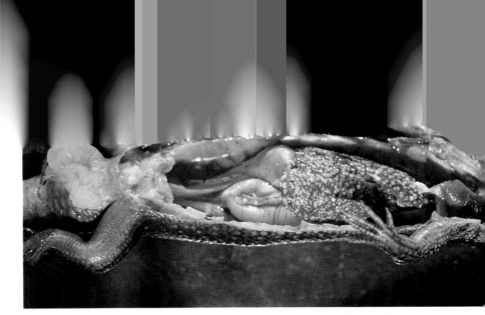

62. Miliary tuberculosis in the liver of an Australian lizard, *Egernia napoleonsis*. The small (miliary) tubercles are still well separated from one another. Photo: Elkan.

63. Leishman stained smear of fish blood showing unidentified bacteria. Photo: Piscisan Ltd.

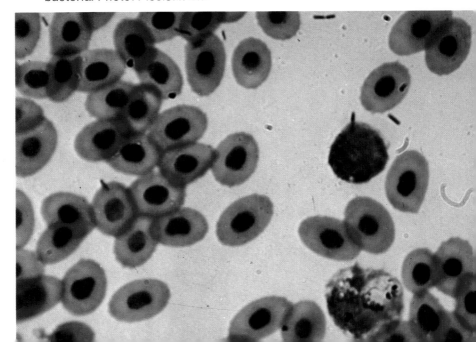

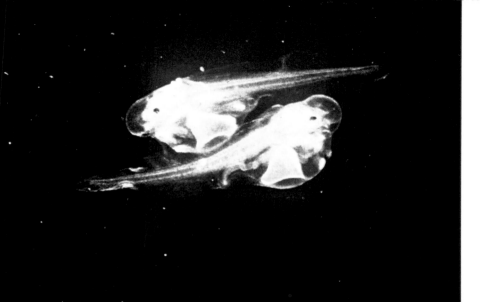

64. *Phractura ansorgei* with dropsy of the yolk sac. This condition is caused mostly by nutritional deficiency and is rarely of bacterial origin. Photo: Foersch.

65-68. These photos show, respectively, *Synodontis petricola* and *Datnioides microlepis* affected with an unidentified bacterial disease. The fish exhibited white necrotic external lesions and granulomata of the internal organs. Photos: Dr. Herbert R. Axelrod.

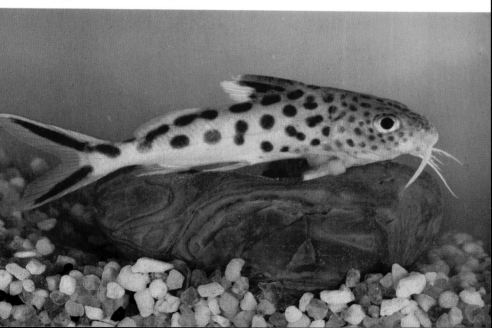

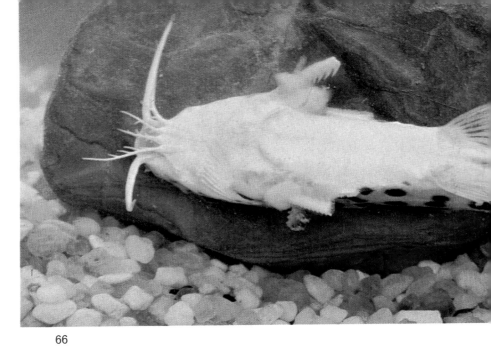

66

67

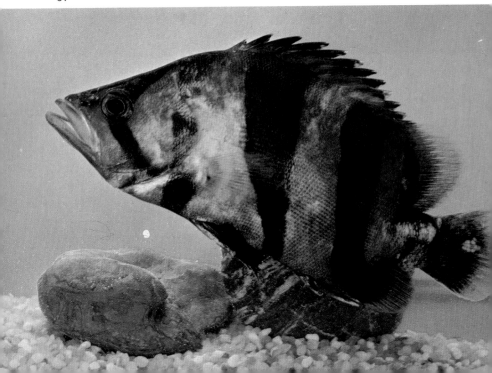

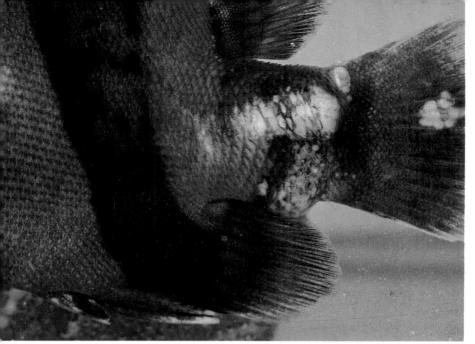

68

69. Histological section through the external lesion of *Datnioides microlepis* showing necrotic tissue debris and remnants of skeletal muscle. Photo: Landolt.

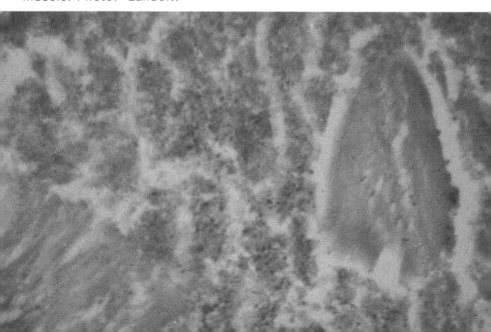

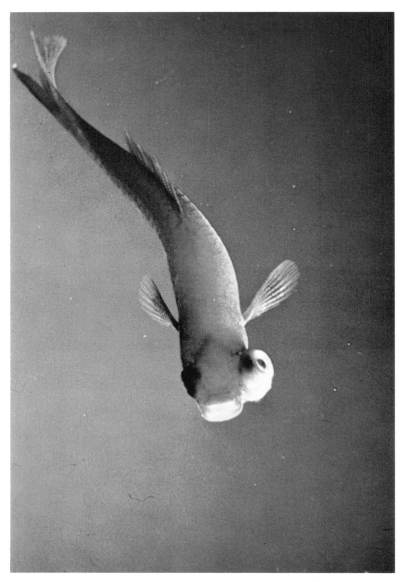

70. Exophthalmos in a swordtail *(Xiphophorus helleri)*. This is a common condition and is often associated with bacterial infections. Photo: Frickhinger.

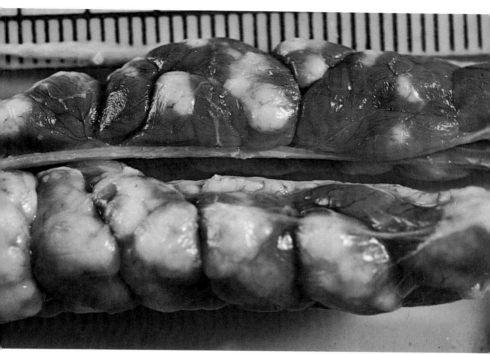

71. Kidney of a Sinai desert cobra *(Walterinnesia aegyptia)*. This snake and several others of the same species died at short intervals after they had thrived well in captivity for several months. Grossly, the lesion resembles a malignant tumor, fungal disease or tuberculosis. None of these diagnoses applied. Apart from the kidneys, the lung and the thyroid gland were found diseased. Granulomata similar to those seen in tuberculosis were found in the affected organs together with foreign body giant cells and Langhans giant cells. There was no caseation or acid fast bacteria. The destruction of the affected organs was almost total. Compared with what is seen in human pathology, the picture nearest to what was seen in these snakes is that of sarcoidosis, but this disease has not been recognized in animals. A systemic granulomatous disease of viral origin is a possibility, and the fact that the disease occurred in the form of an epizootic suggests that it was infectious. Photo: Elkan.

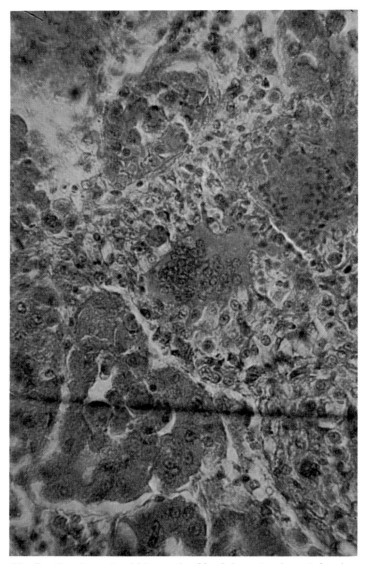

72. Section from the kidney of a Sinai desert cobra stained with a reticulin stain. Note the tubercles with central fibrinoid necrosis and an absence of reticulin pattern. Photo: Elkan.

III. PARASITIC DISEASES

A. Fungi

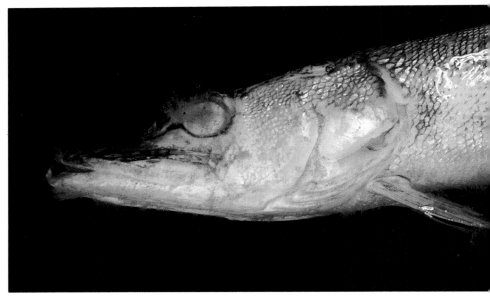

73. Saprolegniasis of pike *(Esox lucius)*.

74. Reddish lesions caused by *Saprolegnia* sp. in a goldfish *(Carassius auratus)*.

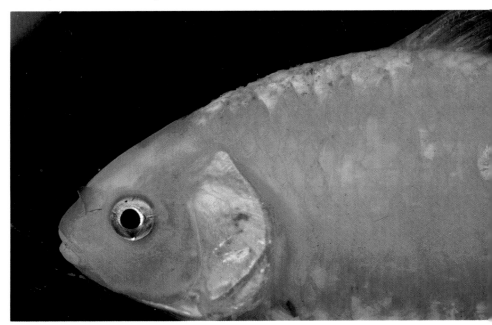

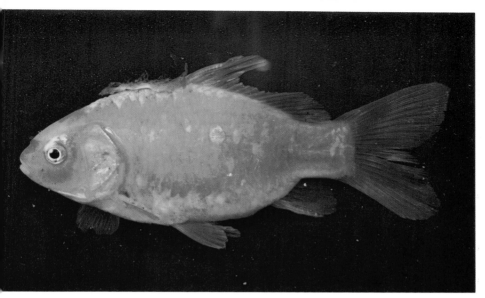

75. *Saprolegnia,* the water mold, on the skin of a fish. Photo: Frickhinger.

76. *Saprolegnia* invading a wound sustained by a common scat *(Scatophagus argus).* Photo: Frickhinger.

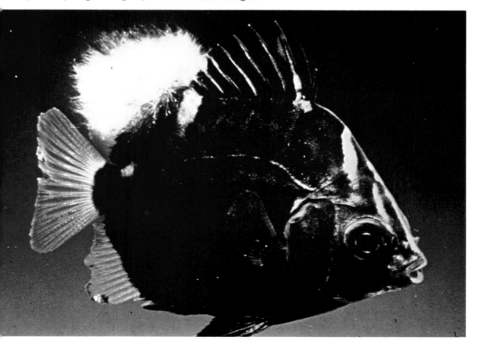

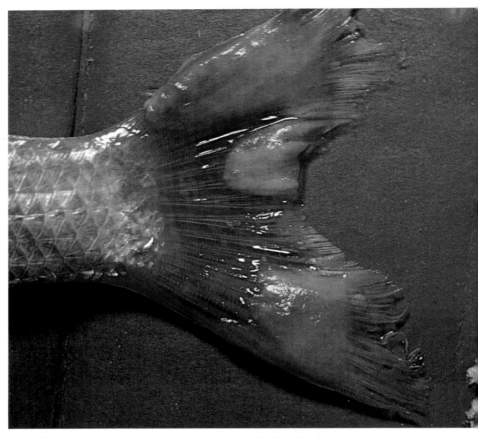

77. Secondary *Saprolegnia* infection of tail rot lesion.

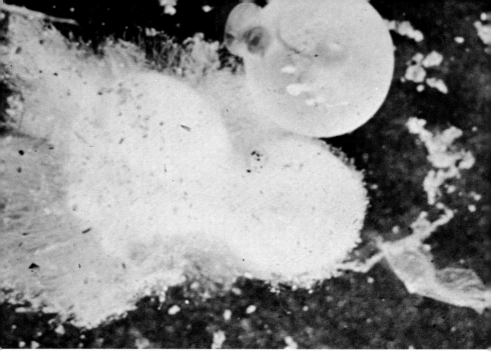

78. Eggs of rainbow trout *(Salmo gairdneri)* attacked by *Saprolegnia.*

79. Achlyiasis and trichodiniasis of salmonid fish.

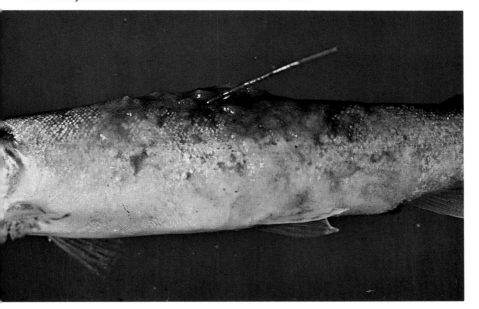

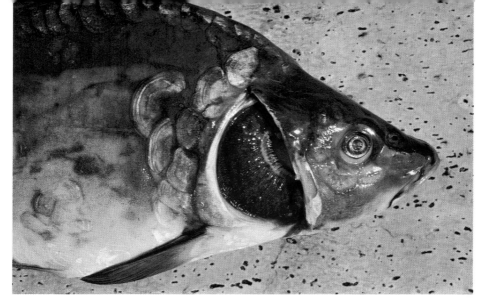

80. Gill rot in a carp caused by the fungus *Branchiomyces.* Photo:
Dr. P. de Kinkelin.

81. Hyphae of *Branchiomyces* in the gills of a pike (*Esox* sp.). Photo:
Frickhinger.

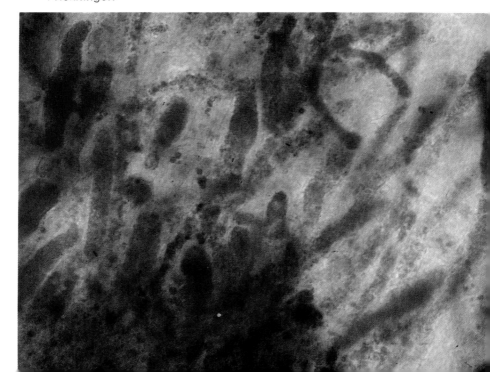

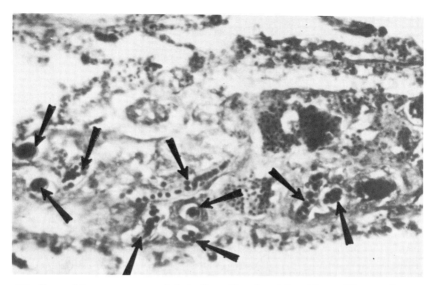

82. *Branchiomyces sanguinis* in the gills of a striped bass *(Roccus).*
The arrows indicate fungal filaments or spores.

83. *Branchiomyces sanguinis* in the gills of a striped bass *(Roccus).*
The arrows indicate fungal filaments.

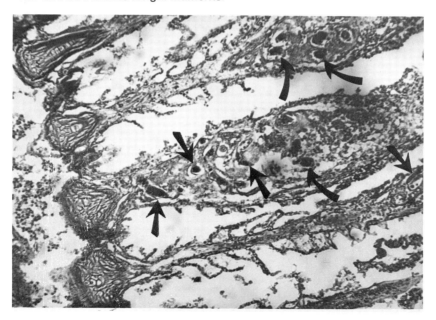

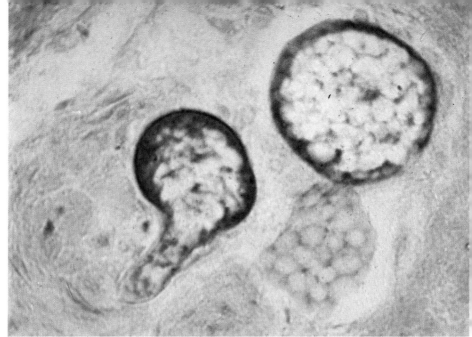

84. Plasmodia of *Ichthyophonus* (formerly *Ichthyosporidium*) *hoferi* emerging from cysts in the liver of a rainbow trout (*Salmo gairdneri*).

85. *Ichthyophonus* is a fungus commonly seen in fish, but it may attack other aquatic animals like newts and frogs. It is usually found in the form of cysts which may change the appearance of the tissue to such an extent that it looks like gruyere cheese. The fungus occurs mainly in marine fish, where it is of economic importance, but it seems equally capable of surviving in fresh water. Photo: Elkan.

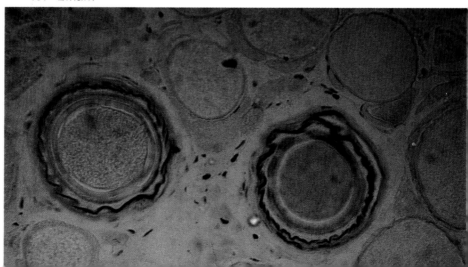

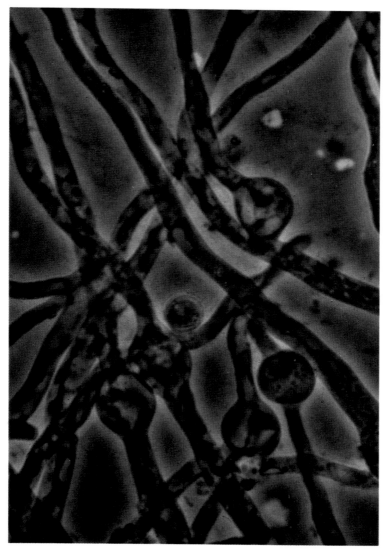

86. *Aphanomyces* sp. taken from *Symphysodon discus*. Photo: Frickhinger.

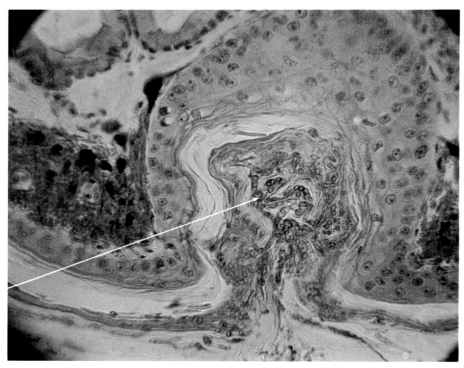

87. Fungi and their spores must be even more ubiquitous in the environment of lower vertebrates than tubercle bacilli, yet cases of fungal infection are not very common either in amphibians or in reptiles. Here we see fungal threads (hyphae) in a recess of the skin of a chameleon, but these fungi may be harmless commensals and remain so until they find an opportunity to breach the skin. They can then become lethal because no tissue can prevent their progress, and they may eventually find their way into the spinal canal and the brain. Photo: Elkan.

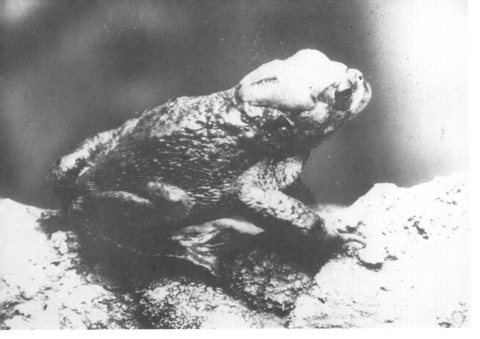

88. A European toad *(Bufo bufo)* with an extensive fungal infection of the skin of the head. The infection had not yet reached the brain, and the toad behaved normally. Photo: Elkan.

89. This large ulcer on *Smilisca baudini* proved to be due to a fungal infection. Photo: Elkan.

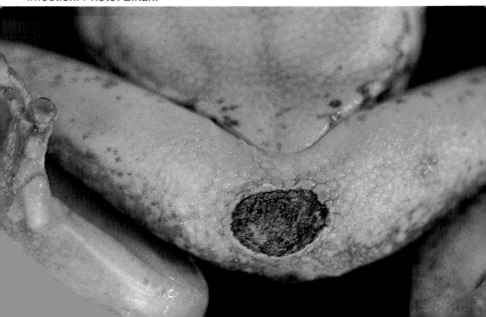

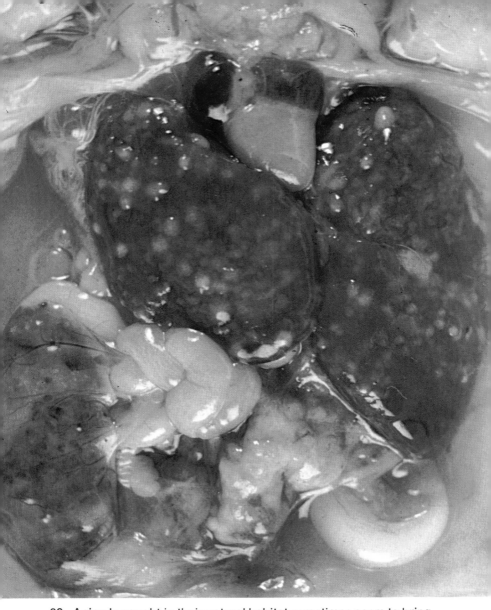

90. Animals caught in their natural habitat sometimes seem to bring
the seeds of future disaster with them, and it can happen that whole
collections of valuable amphibians are wiped out by fungal epidemics.
Since we cannot assume that all the frogs in one collection suffer skin
injuries at the same time which would give access to fungi, these
must somehow gain admittance through the natural apertures of the
body, probably through the lungs and/or the stomach. The North
American tree frog *(Hyla cinerea)* in this photograph showed no
external lesion, but it had extensive mycosis of the liver. Photo: Elkan.

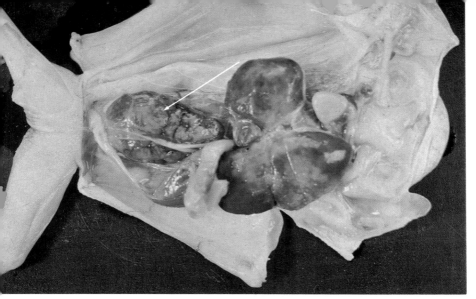

91. Another specimen from the epizootic described in figure 90 shows fungal invasion of the intestine. Photo: Elkan.

92. Microscopically a fungus can present many different forms. In all its shapes it can be found either lying free in normal or in necrotic tissue or taken up by large multinucleated cells which seem to make an attempt at destroying the fungus. This picture shows a fungal thread ending in a terminal spore. Photo: Elkan.

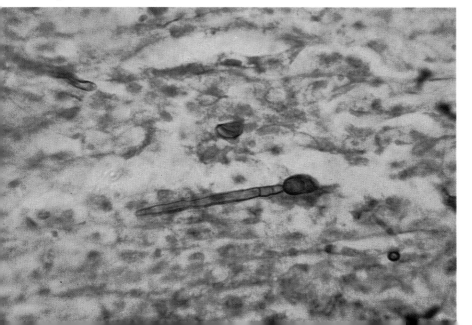

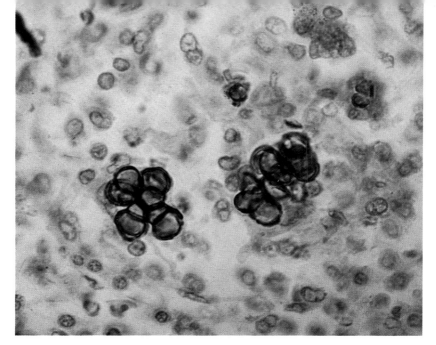

93. Clusters of fungal spores. Photo: Elkan.

94. Occasionally, if the fungal infestation is very heavy, several giant cells may combine in the attack, forming a syncytium. The fungus, however, seems to be quite unaffected by these attempts to destroy it. Photo: Elkan.

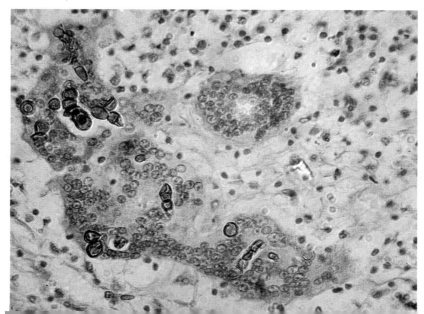

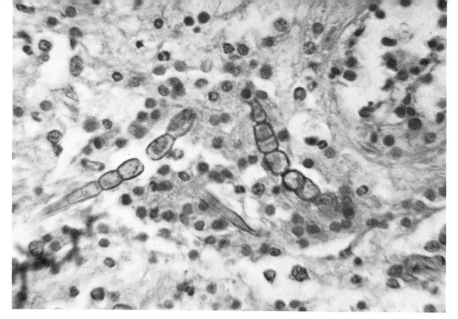

95. A giant cell attempting to destroy a chain of fungal spores.
Photo: Elkan.

96. In this picture a giant cell is shown which has engulfed some
fungal elements but has in the process become damaged to such an
extent that its nuclei have become pycnotic (clumped). These nuclei
do not recover. The prognosis once a fungus has established itself in
an amphibian is always hopeless. Photo: Elkan.

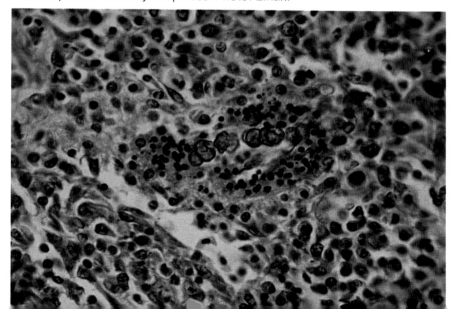

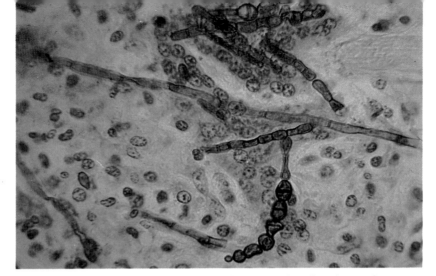

97. Detail from a fungal granuloma in *Hyla caerulea* showing a giant cell in the process of engulfing mycelial threads. We never see any evidence that these threads are actually digested by the giant cells. The cells, composed of the confluence of many monocytes, react to the presence of a foreign body but are unable to destroy or even to damage it. Photo: Elkan.

98. This North American corn snake *(Elaphe guttata)* was kept in a cage for several years before it developed a soft tumor in the region of the neck. Since the snake seemed otherwise healthy, surgical removal of the tumor was attempted. Photo: Elkan.

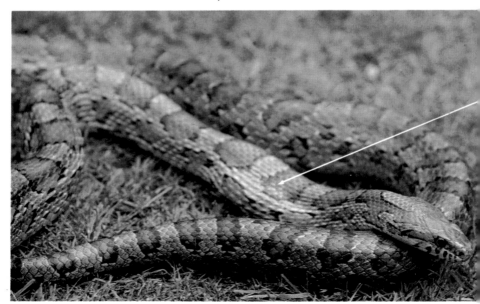

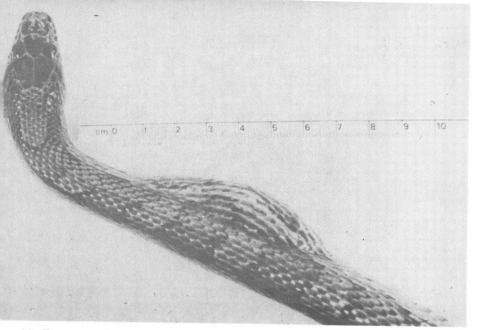

99. The operation was successfully performed at the London Zoo Hospital (Mr. J. F. Hime). The tumor, which lay between the skin and the cervical viscera, was found to be due to fungal invasion. The snake recovered quickly. Photo: Elkan.

100. If a fungus gains entrance between the bone and scale of a turtle carapace, the scales may become detached. Since the bone presents an obstacle to any further progress of the fungus, the animal itself is not affected, but the scales are never replaced. The turtle in the picture is *Testudo hermanni*. Photo: Elkan.

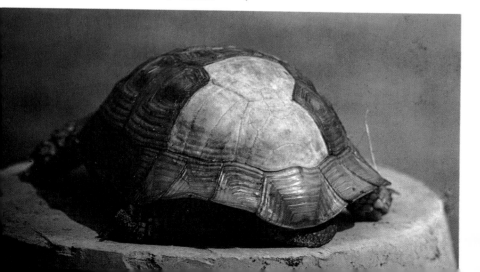

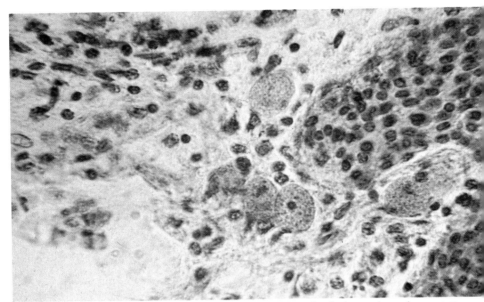

101-102.   *Chameleo   dilepis*, the flap-necked chameleon, is a common African lizard. *Amoeba invadens* is a protozoan similar to *Amoeba histolytica*, which produces severe ulcerative colitis and liver abscesses in man. The organisms shown in figures 101-102 were found during examination of a papillomatous growth which had formed around the cloaca of the chameleon. The anal passage seemed obstructed through edema and inflammation. The animal refused to feed and died either from inanition or from toxic products produced by the amebae. Both causes may have been contributory. Photos: Elkan.

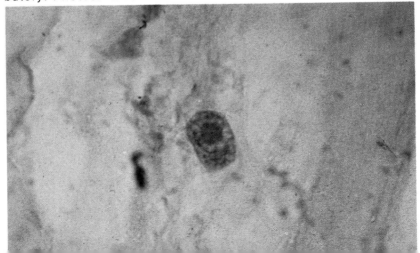

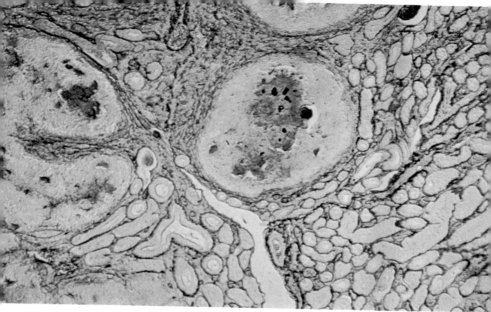

103. Amebae of the *histolytica* type are usually found in the lower intestine where they cause inflammation, ulceration and occasionally abscess formation in the liver. The remarkable feature of the case here illustrated is that the amebae were found in the connective tissue surrounding labial glands and in the dermis. There were no signs of any defensive reaction on the part of the host lizard *(Ptyodactylus hasselquisti)*. Amebae in tissue are best demonstrated by using a Giemsa stain. Photo: Elkan.

104. *Amoeba invadens* in an Israeli gecko *(Ptyodactylus hasselquisti)*. Photo: Elkan.

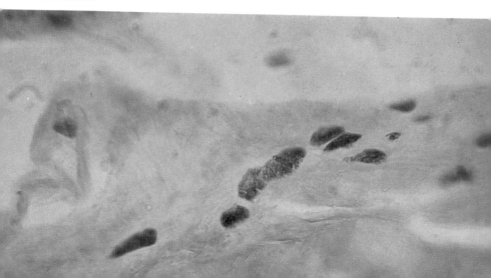

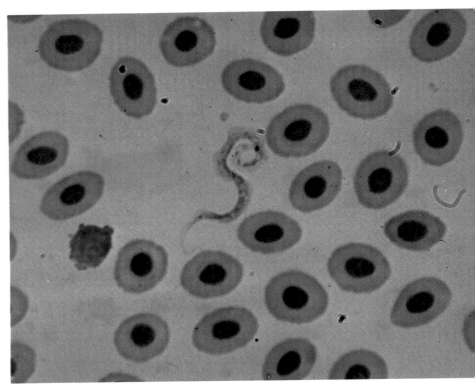

105. *Trypanosoma sp.* in the blood of a European eel (*Anguilla anguilla*). Photo: Piscisan Ltd.

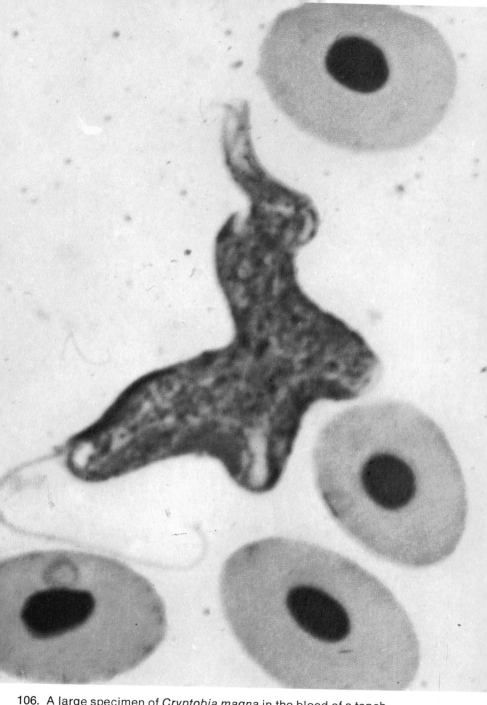

106. A large specimen of *Cryptobia magna* in the blood of a tench
(Tinca tinca).

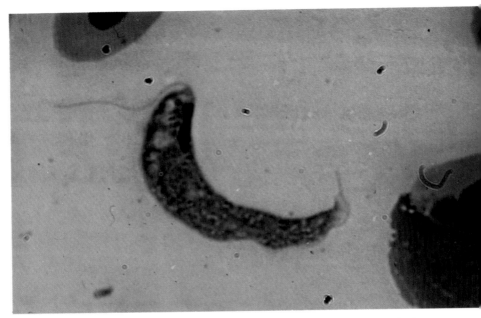

107. *Cryptobia* sp. in the blood of an Atlantic salmon *(Salmo salar)* parr.

108. *Costia necatrix* on a brown trout *(Salmo trutta).*

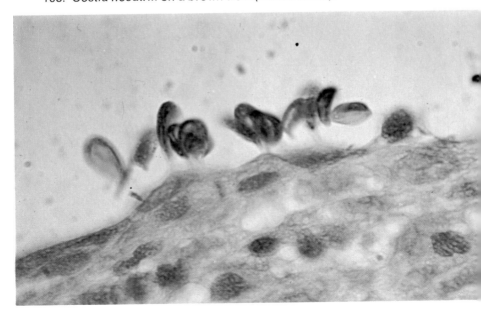

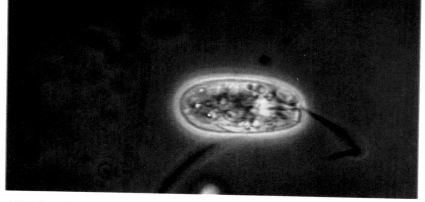

109. *Costia necatrix,* a unicellular flagellate parasite of the skin and the gills. The parasite attaches itself to the skin, where it feeds on skin debris and causes dark patches to appear. Costiasis, due to abundant infestation, can cause mass mortality. Photo: Frickhinger.

110. A discus fish *(Symphysodon discus)* heavily infected with *Hexamita.* Note the damage to the head. Photo: Frickhinger.

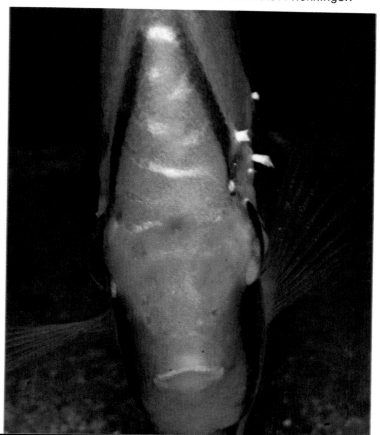

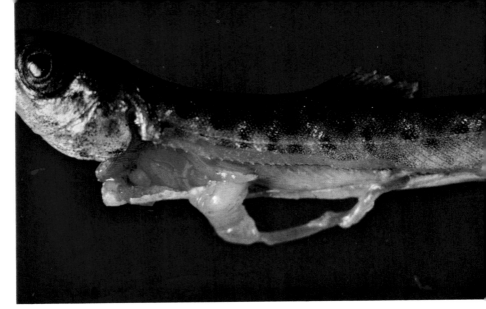

111. Hexamitiasis in rainbow trout *(Salmo gairdneri)*.

112. *Hexamita intestinalis,* a unicellular parasite in the peritoneal fluid of a discus fish *(Symphysodon discus).* The parasite lives in body fluids, the blood, the intestine and the skin where it may cause severe damage. Photo: Frickhinger.

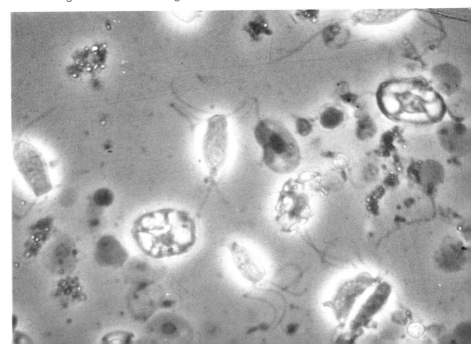

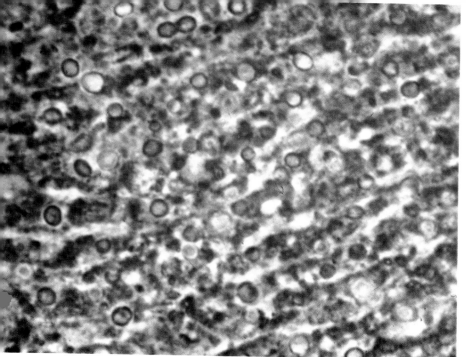

113. *Oodinioides vastator*, a unicellular flagellate parasite causing white dermal discoloration. Note the prominent dinospores. Photo: Frickhinger.

114. Sporulating stage of *Oodinioides vastator*. Photo: Frickhinger.

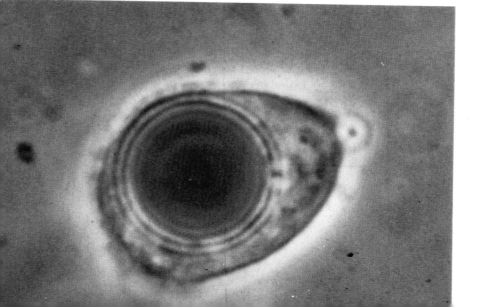

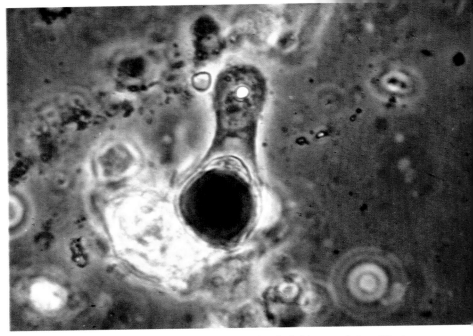

115. Plasmodium with sporangium of *Oodinioides vastator.* Photo: Frickhinger.

116. *Oodinioides vastator* attached to the gills of a fish. Photo: Frickhinger.

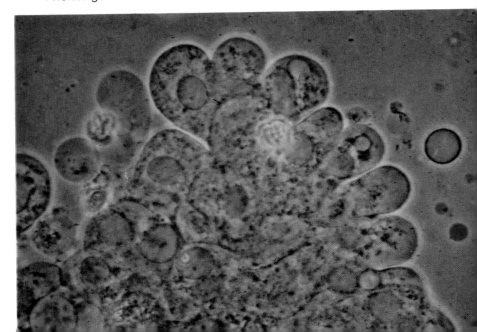

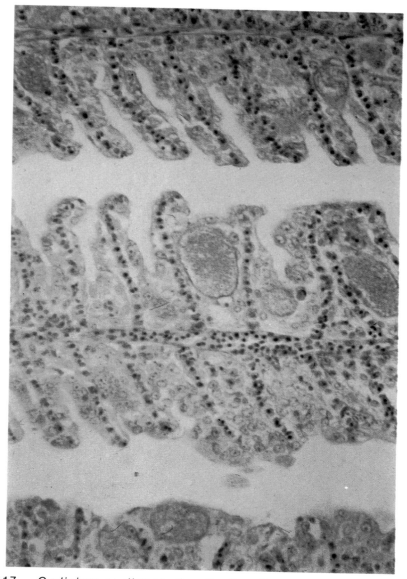

117. *Oodinium ocellatum*, the dinoflagellate causing velvet, attached to the gills of a coral fish.

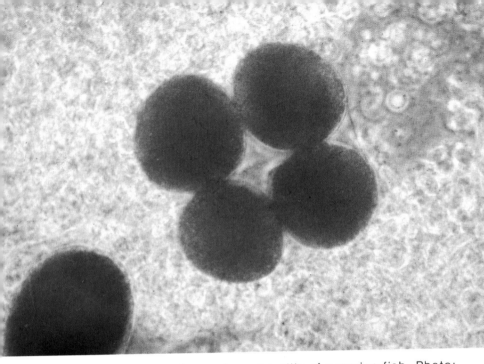

118. *Oodinium ocellatum* from the gills of a marine fish. Photo: Frickhinger.

119. *Oodinioides vastator.* Sporulating stage. Photo: Frickhinger.

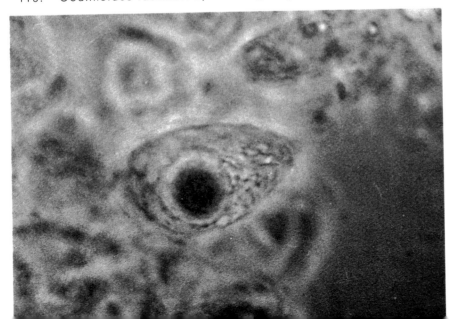

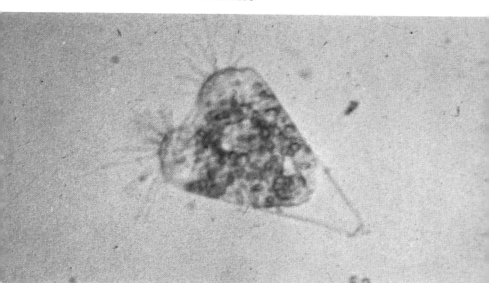

120.   *Trichophrya piscium* , an ectoparasitic sessile ciliate. Photo: Reichenbach-Klinke.

121.   Large white spots in the skin of an angelfish caused by *Cryptocaryon*, which lives embedded in the skin. Photo: Frickhinger.

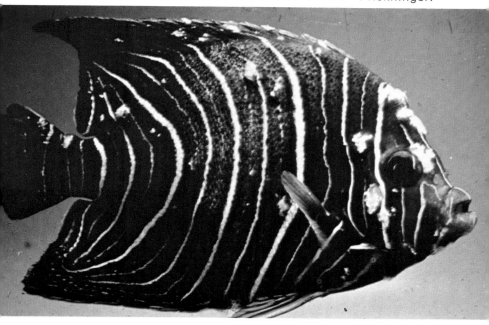

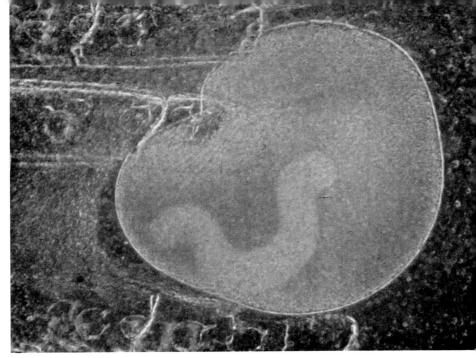

122. A solitary specimen of *Cryptocaryon* sp. Photo: Frickhinger.

123. A juvenile barb *(Barbus* species) with white-spot disease caused by a unicellular ciliate, *Ichthyophthirius multifilis.* The parasite invades the skin of fishes and encapsulates. Each white spot contains one parasite. Photo: Frickhinger.

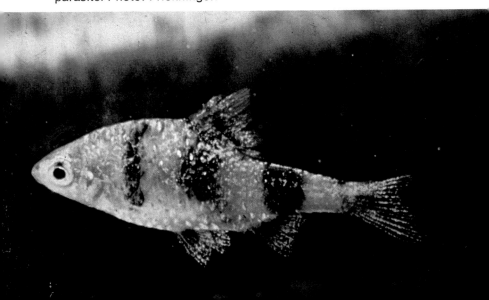

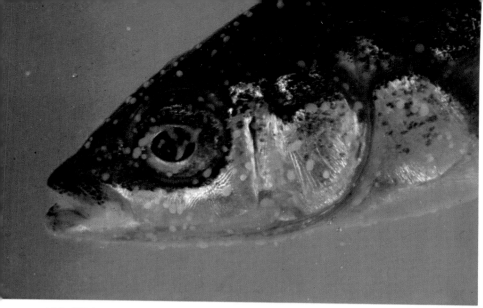

124. White spot *(Ichthyophthirius)* in three-spined stickleback *(Gasterosteus aculeatus)*.

125. White spot disease *(Ichthyophthirius)* in the false featherback *(Xenomystus niger)*. Photo: Frickhinger.

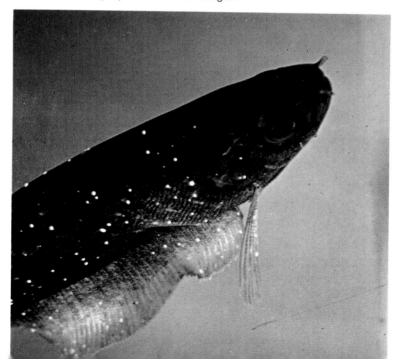

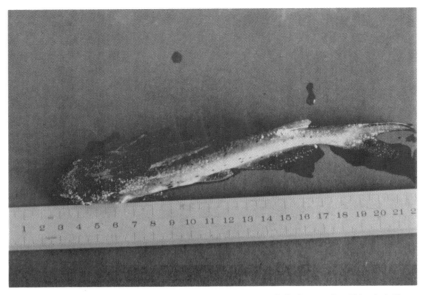

126. Channel catfish (*Ictalurus punctatus*) infected with *Ichthyophthirius multifilis*.

127. *Ichthyophthirius* in the fin of a channel catfish.

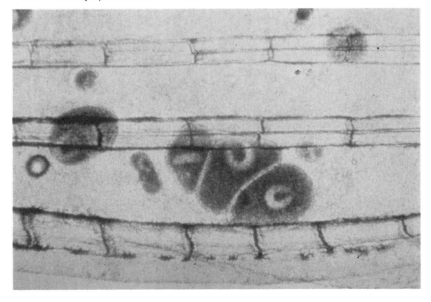

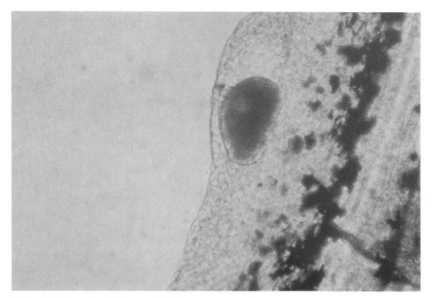

128. *Ichthyophthirius multifilis* embedded in the fin of a channel catfish *(Ictalurus punctatus)*.

129. This photograph shows a single *Ichthyophthirius multifilis* embedded in the pseudobranch (part of the gill system) of the fish *(Scardinius erythrophthalmus)*. The parasite is harmless if it occurs in small numbers. Photo: Elkan.

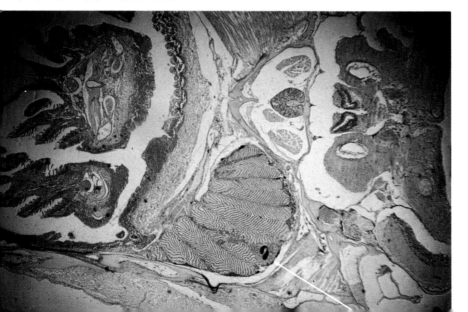

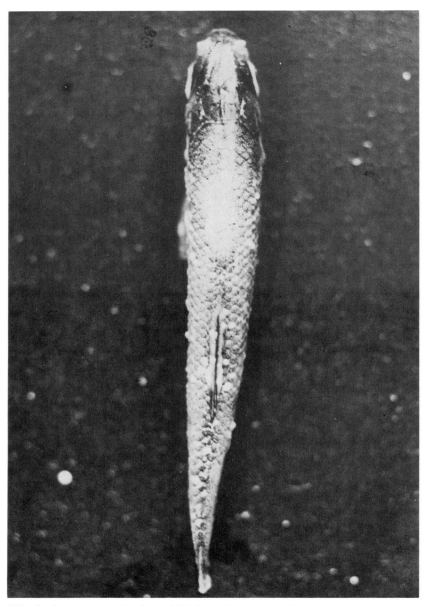

130. Unfortunately, *Ichthyophthirius* often occurs in very large numbers and may then cause debility or even the death of the fish. Photo: Elkan.

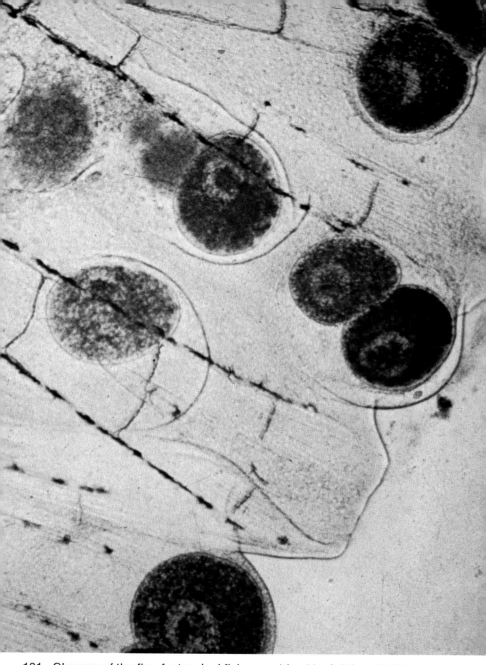

131. Closeup of the fin of a tropical fish parasitized by *Ichthyophthirius multifilis.* Photo: Frickhinger.

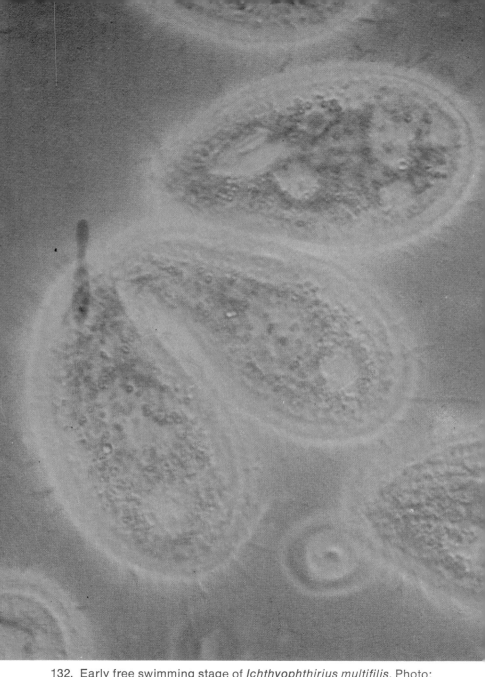

132. Early free swimming stage of *Ichthyophthirius multifilis*. Photo: Frickhinger.

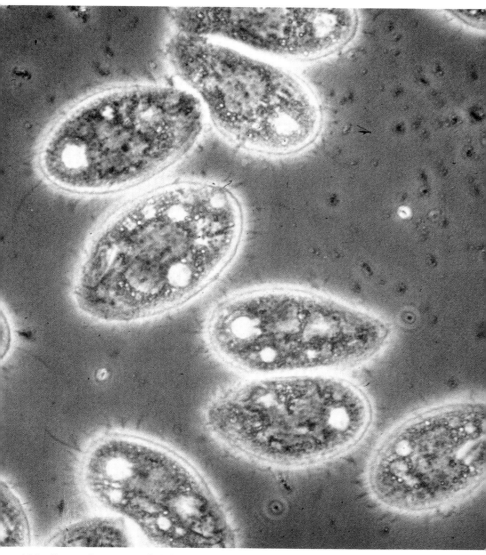

133. Swarming young *Ichthyophthirius multifilis*. Photo: Frickhinger.

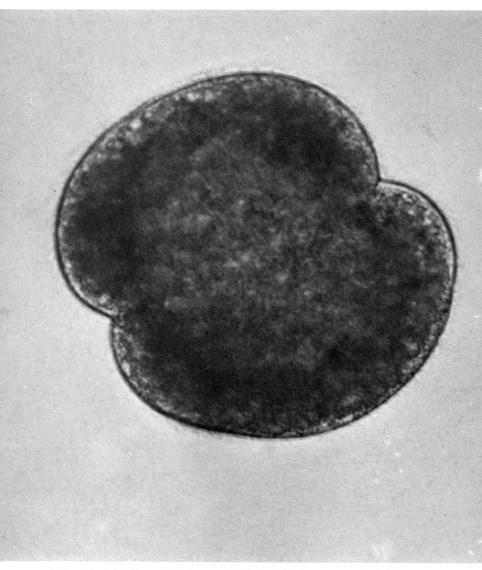

134. Adult *Ichthyophthirius multifilis* in initial process of division.
Photo: Frickhinger.

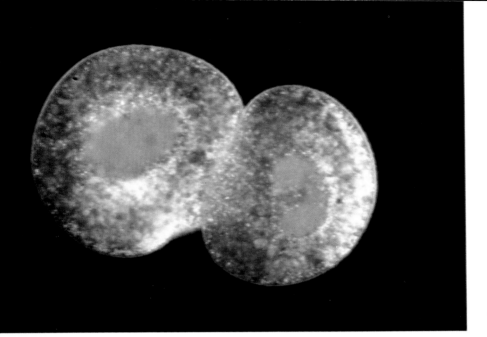

135. Adult *Ichthyophthirius multifilis* dividing into two cells. Photo: Frickhinger.

136. Adult *Ichthyophthirius multifilis*.

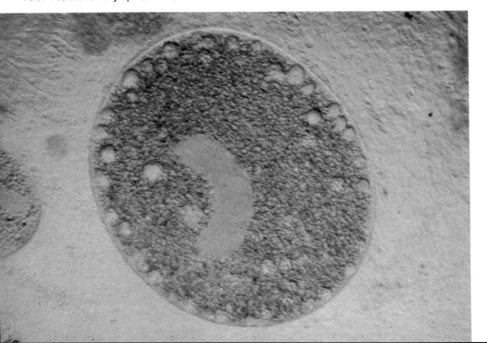

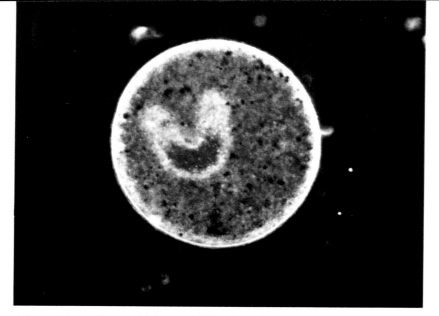

137. Adult *Ichthyophthirius multifilis.* Note the horseshoe-shaped nucleus. Photo: Frickhinger.

138. *Tetrahymena* sp., a facultative parasite that occasionally infects fish. Photo: Frickhinger.

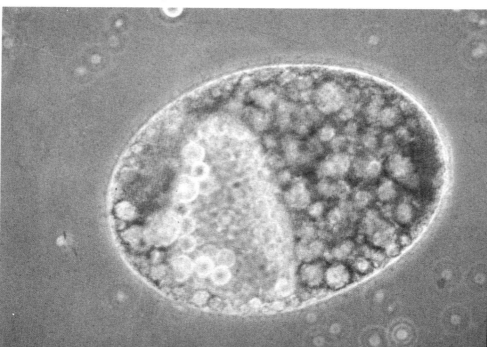

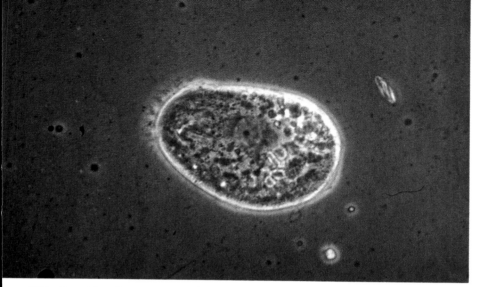

139. *Brooklynella* sp., a parasite similar to *Tetrahymena* but limited to marine waters. Photo: Frickhinger.

140. *Balantidium* sp., an oblong ciliate which parasitizes the gills of fish. Photo: Frickhinger.

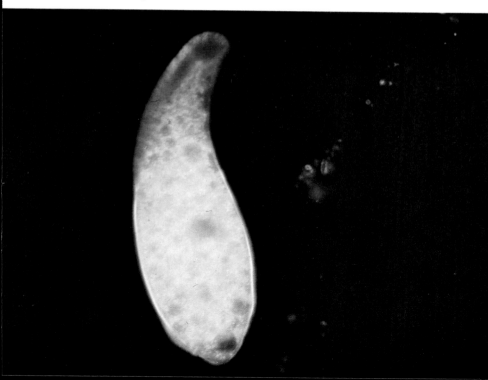

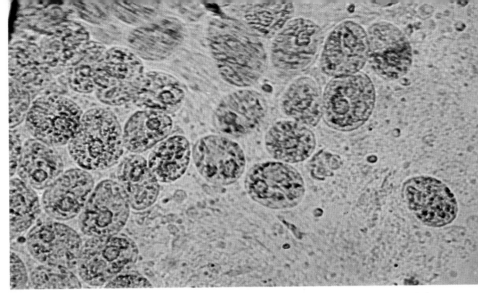

141. Juvenile forms of *Chilodonella* sp. from the gills of a tropical fish.

142. *Chilodonella cyprini*, a unicellular parasite from the gills of a carp. If abundant, the parasite causes grey discoloration of the skin, hence, it is often called "the great skin darkener." Note the striations.

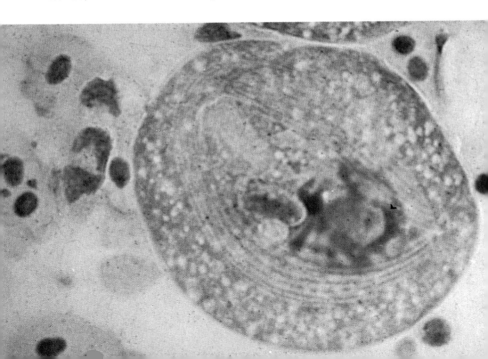

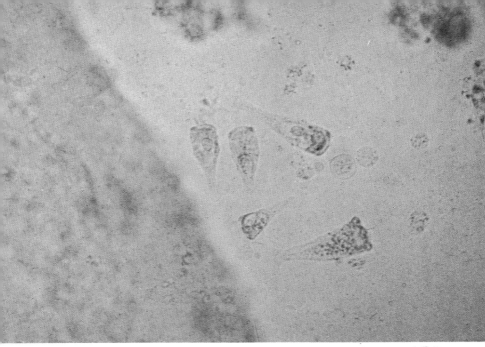

143. *Apiosoma* (formerly *Glossatella*) *piscicola* taken from a carp. Photo: Reichenbach-Klinke.

144. *Trichodinella* sp., an ectoparasite of fish. These parasites are unicellular. They move about on the surface of the fish, feeding on cell debris. Photo: Frickhinger.

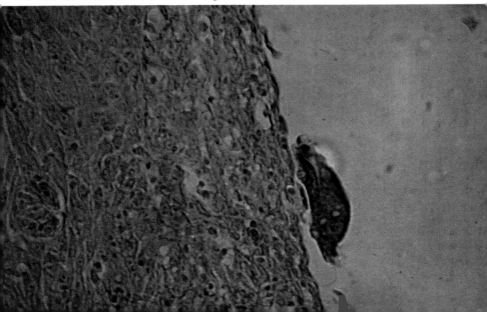

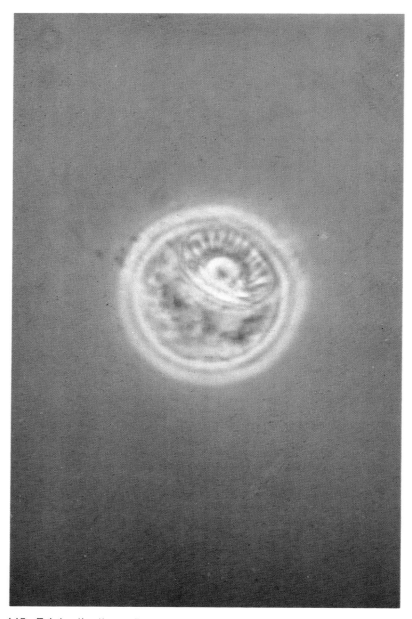

145. *Trichodinella* sp. Photo: Frickhinger.

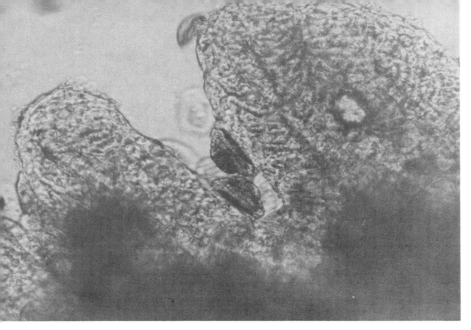

146. Infestation of *Trichodina sp.* on goldfish *Carassius auratus.*
Photo: Frank Leteaux, Ozark Fisheries Inc.

147. *Trichodina* sp. Photo: Frickhinger.

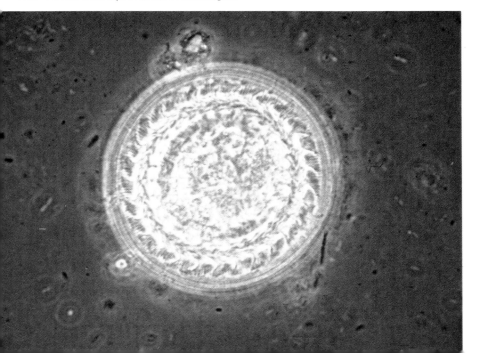

d. Sporozoans

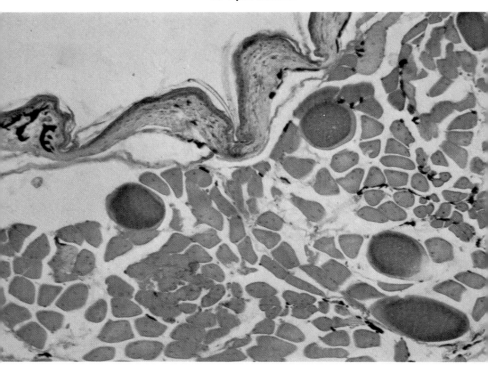

148. *Sarcocystis* is a protozoan which still puzzles the protozoologists. It has not even been definitely established whether this parasite might, in fact, be a fungus. It is found in the muscle fibers of vertebrates of all kinds, where it spreads along the length of the fibers, forming the so-called Miescher's tubes. A thin external margin of sarcolemma (muscle fiber substance) always remains. The tubes are usually filled with hematoxyphil spores visible only with the aid of high magnification. The complete life cycle of this parasite is not yet known. There is no sign of any defence reaction on the part of the host. The cysts in this photograph were found in the *longissimus dorsi* muscle of an Israeli lizard *(Eremias olivieri)*. Photo: Elkan.

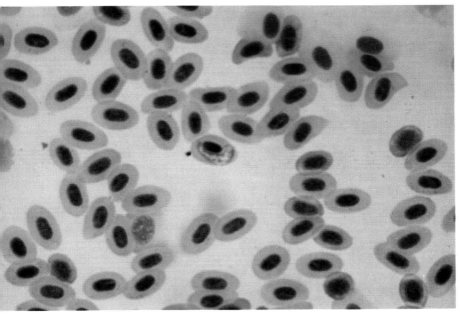

149. Hemogregarine within an erythrocyte of an Atlantic salmon *(Salmo salar)*.

150. Hemogregarines in a reptile. Note the asexual schizogeny, i.e., the production of oblong daughter cells by simple division.

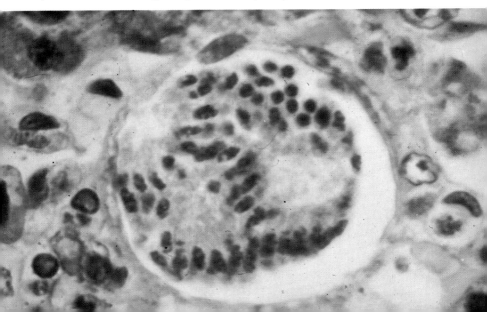

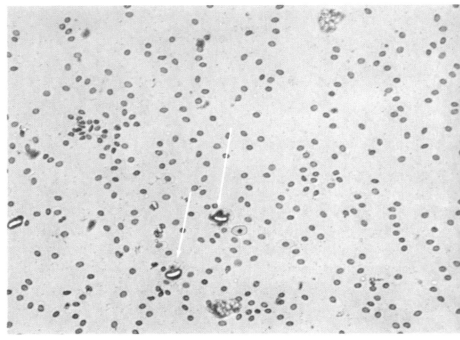

151. Hemogregarines, a type of unicellular blood parasite, in the dabb lizard *(Uromastix* sp.).

152. *Eimeria* sp. in the intestinal epithelium of a fish.

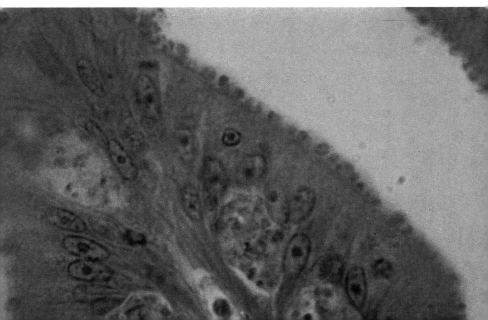

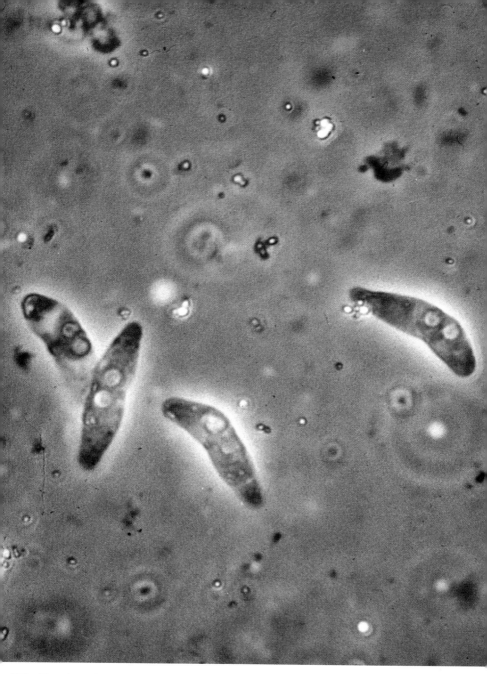

153. Trophozoites of *Ceratomyxa* sp. with ripening spores taken from the gall bladder of *Pomacanthus arcuatus*. Photo: Frickhinger.

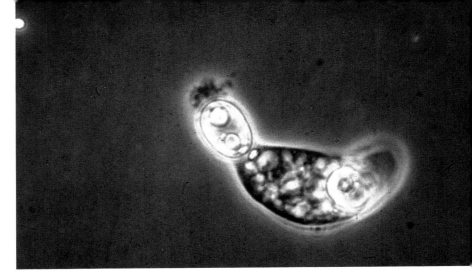

154. Plasmodial stages and spores of *Ceratomyxa* sp., a sporozoan parasite of fish. Photo: Frickhinger.

155. Myxosporidia, unicellular organisms with a complicated life cycle, are more commonly found in fish than in terrestrial forms. *Myxobolus* sp., if it occurs in frogs, displays a predilection for the testes, where it forms large cysts filled with the parasite. The cysts compress the remaining testicular tissue, but apart from possibly interfering with fertility, it is doubtful if the infestation affects the animal as a whole. This photograph shows a *Myxobolus* sp. infestation of *Bufo regularis*. Photo: Elkan.

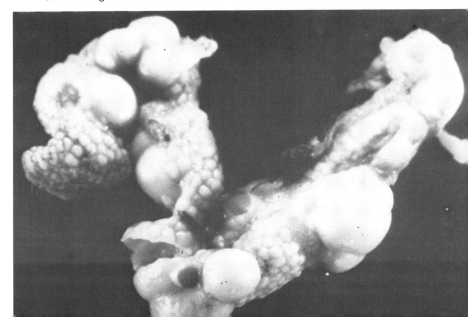

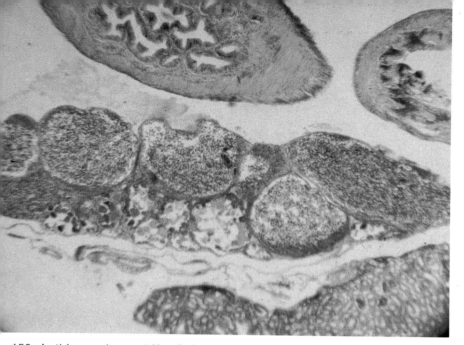

156. In this specimen of *Nyctimistes daymani* only the testes were
found to be affected by the myxosporidian cysts. The frog was caught
in New Guinea and was, so far as is known, not severely affected by
the almost total destruction of the testes. Photo: Elkan.

157. *Myxobolus* sp. from the testis of *Nyctimistes daymani*.
Photo: Elkan.

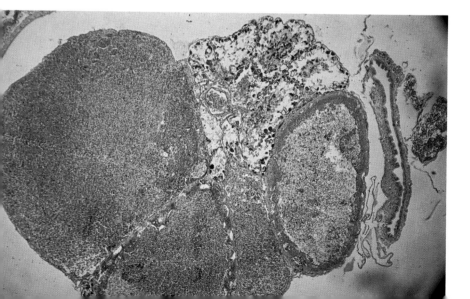

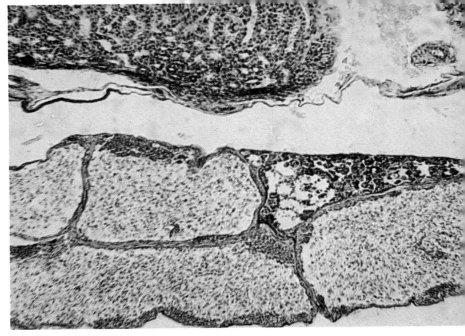

158. *Myxobolus* sp. from the testis of *Nyctimistes daymani.*
Photo: Elkan.

159. *Myxobolus* sp. from the testis of *Nyctimistes daymani* at higher power. Typical of this parasite are the two polar capsules and the iodinophilous vacuole. Photo: Elkan.

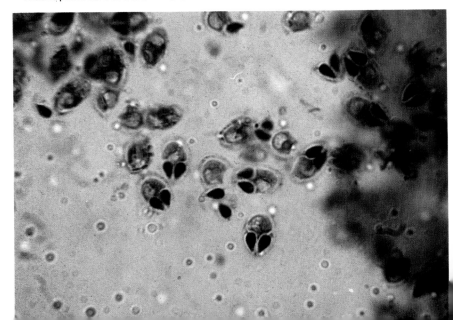

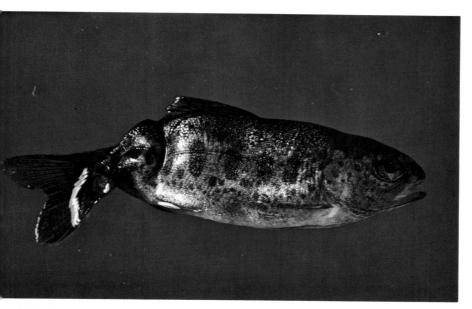

160. Skeletal deformity in rainbow trout (*Salmo gairdneri*) affected with whirling disease caused by *Myxosoma cerebralis.*

161. "Pug nose" in a rainbow trout *(Salmo gairdneri)* that has whirling disease.

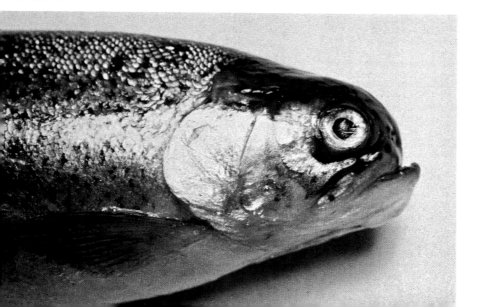

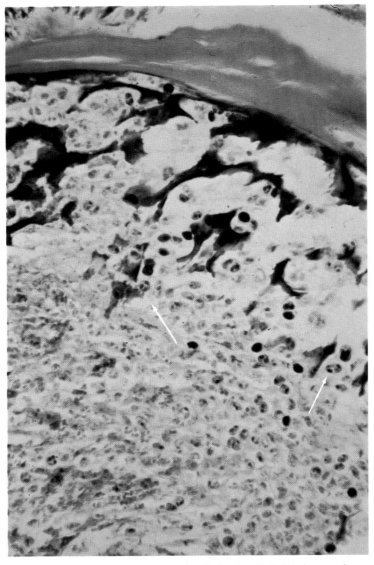

162. Spores of *Myxosoma cerebralis* in the skeletal tissue of a salmonid fish.

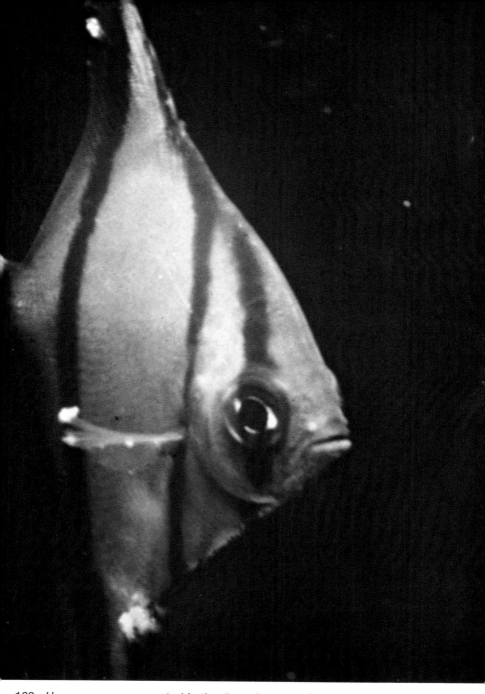

163. *Henneguya* sp. encysted in the fins of a mono *(Monodactylus
sebae).* Photo: Frickhinger.

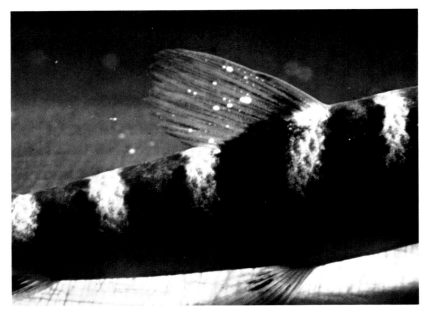

164. Cysts of *Henneguya* sp. on the dorsal fin of *Leporinus* sp.
Photo: Frickhinger.

165. Cutaneous form of *Henneguya* sp. in a channel catfish
(Ictalurus punctatus).

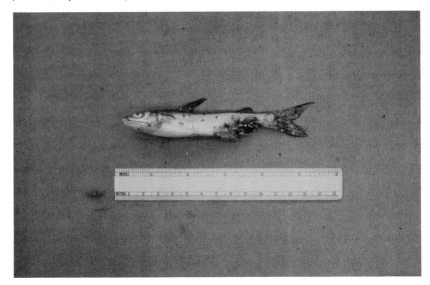

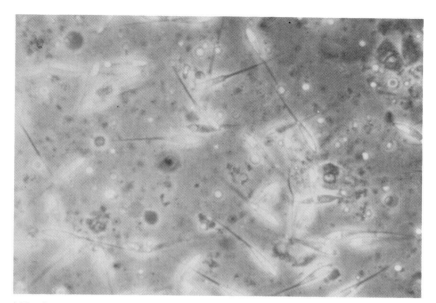

166. Spores of *Henneguya* sp. taken from a channel catfish
(Ictalurus punctatus).

167. Cysts of *Henneguya psorospermica* in the gills of a pike
(Esox lucius). Photo: Dr. P. de Kinkelin.

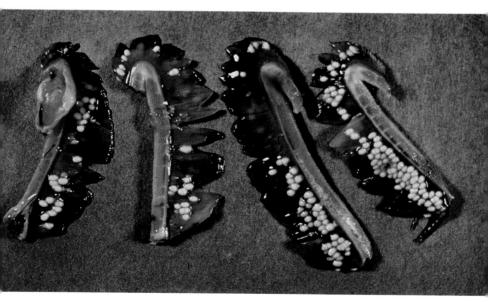

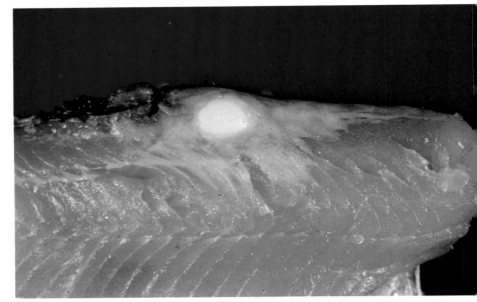

168. Cyst of *Henneguya zschokkei* in the muscle of *Coregonus albula*.

169. Spores of *Henneguya* sp. from a climbing perch (*Ctenopoma* sp.).
Photo: Frickhinger.

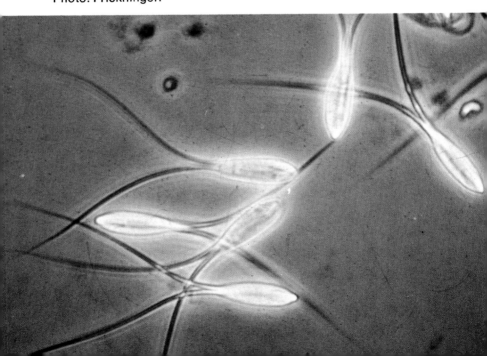

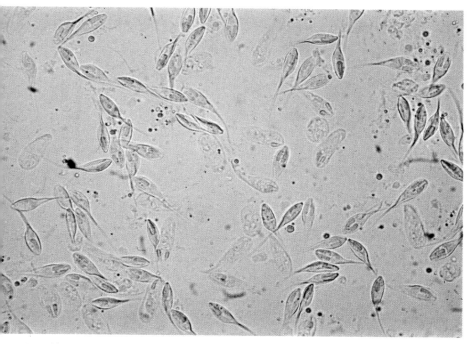

170. *Henneguya psorospermica* from a pike *(Esox lucius)*.

171. Spores of *Henneguya zschokkei*.

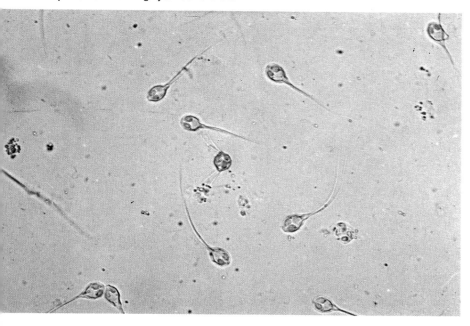

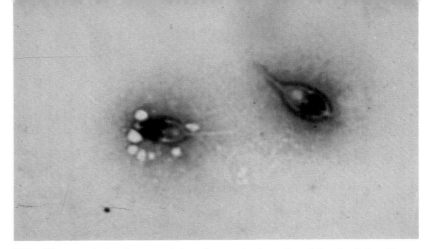

172. Giemsa stained smear taken from a boil on the skin of a fish with myxosporidiasis.

173. The genus *Glugea* belongs to the Microsporidia, very small protozoa which commonly infect fish, particularly the stickleback (*Gasterosteus* sp.), where they produce white cysts in the skin which can easily be seen with the naked eye. This picture shows a fish infected with both *Glugea* sp. and *Schistocephalus* sp. The cysts may severely disfigure the fish and probably hamper its movements, but they do not kill the victim. Occasionally ponds may be found where every fish is infected by *Glugea* sp. Photo: Elkan.

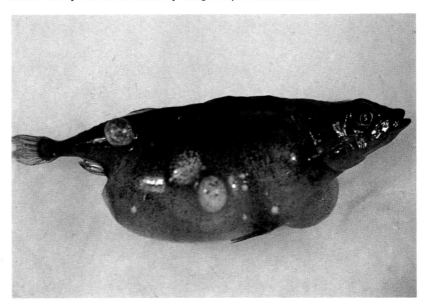

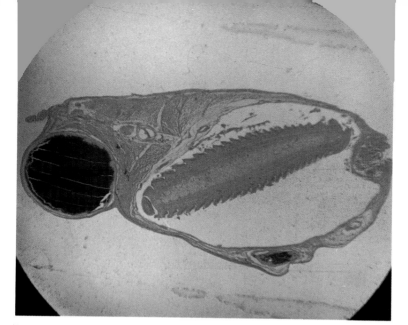

174. Photomicrograph of *Gasterosteus aculeatus* infected with *Glugea* sp. and *Schistocephalus* sp. Photo: Elkan.

175. Cysts of *Glugea anomala* on a three-spined stickleback (*Gasterosteus aculeatus*).

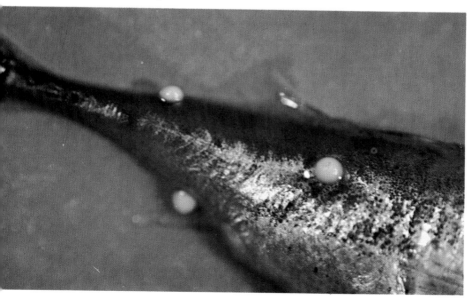

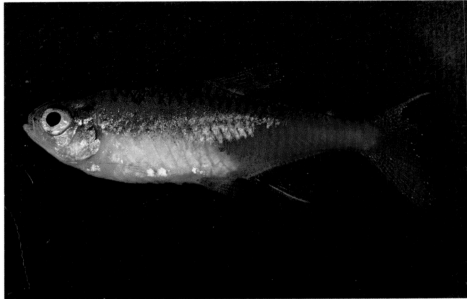

176. Neon tetra (*Paracheirodon innesi*) infected with *Plistophora hyphessobryconis*. This is a microsporidian parasite of the musculature. Photo: Frickhinger.

177. Pansporoblast stage of *Plistophora* taken from a neon tetra. Photo: Frickhinger.

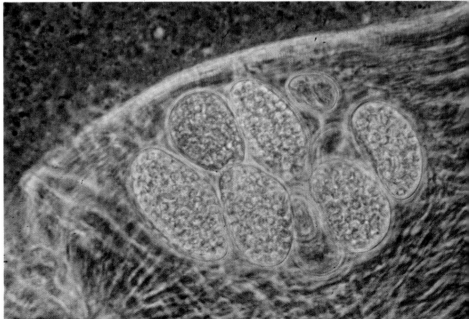

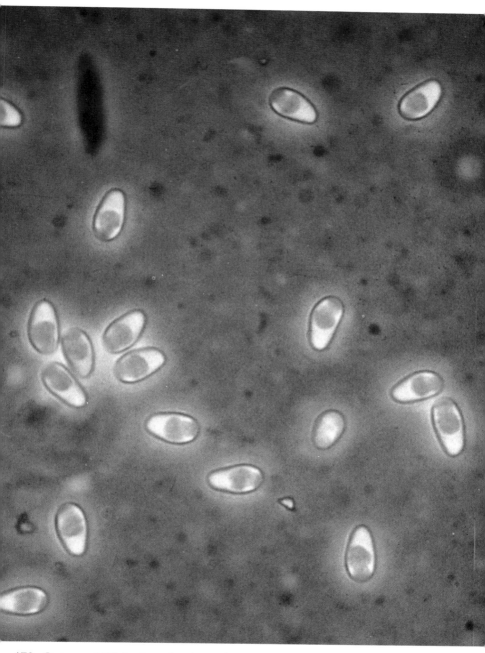

178. Spores of *Plistophora hyphessobryconis* taken from a neon tetra *(Paracheirodon innesi)*. Photo: Frickhinger.

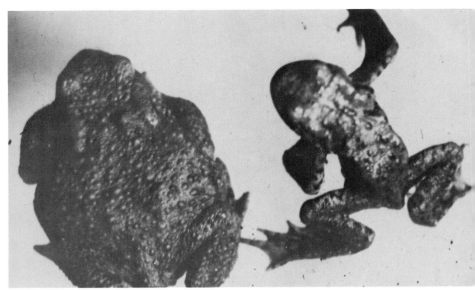

179. An epizootic due to infection with a microsporidian occurred in a population of European common toads *(Bufo bufo)* in southern England. The picture shows a normal toad (left) and another affected by the development of the parasite in its skeletal muscle. Photo: Elkan.

180. This microsporidian develops in and destroys the muscle fibers. Naked-eye inspection shows the long white streaks following the direction of the frog's muscles. Photo: Elkan.

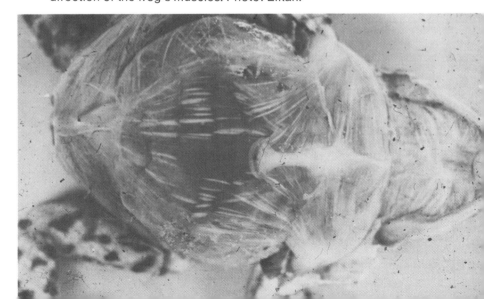

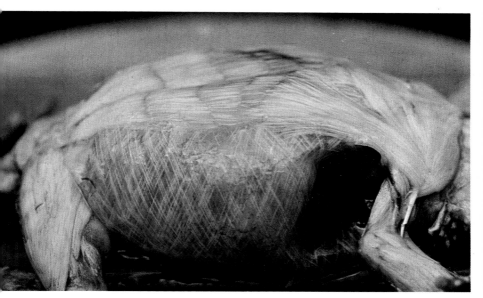

181-182. These figures show the lateral abdominal wall where the fibers of two sheets of muscles (internal and external obliques) cross; the parasitic cysts cross accordingly. Photos: Elkan.

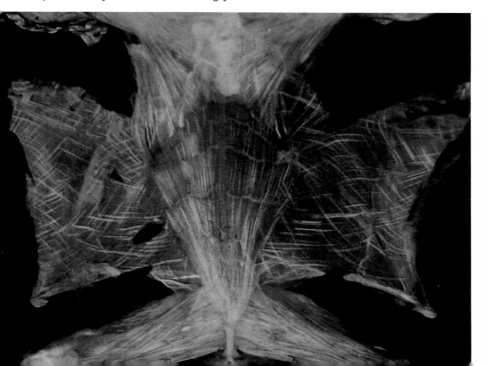

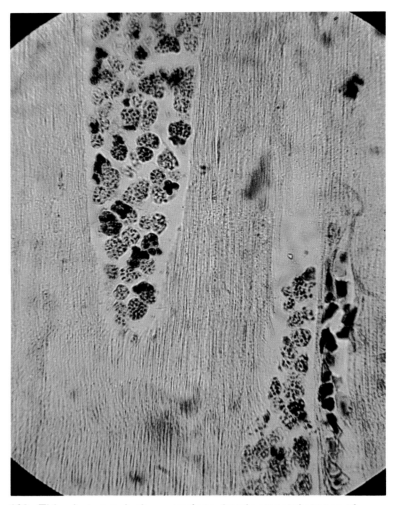

183. This photograph shows various developmental stages of *Plistophora myotrophica* in the muscle fibers of *Bufo bufo.*
Photo: Elkan.

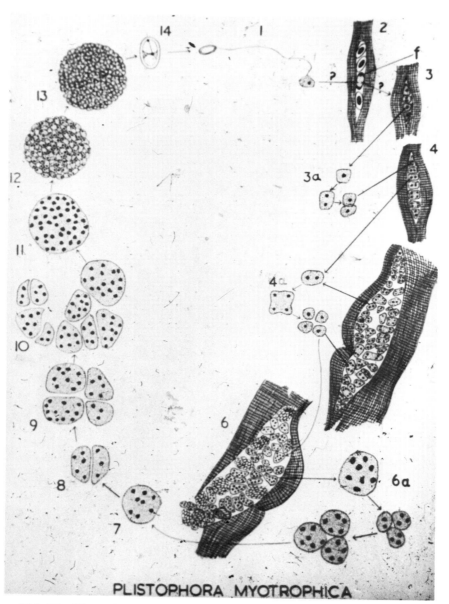

184. The life cycle of *Plistophora myotrophica*.

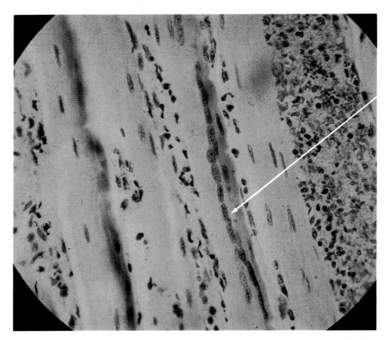

185. A feature very rarely seen is the development of long chains of muscle cells which consist only of nuclei and have practically no cytoplasm. Pictures of this kind occur only in heavily infected toads whose skeletal muscle has been severely damaged by the microsporidian *Plistophora myotrophica*. As a repair process, the development of these nuclear chains is never successful. Photo: Elkan.

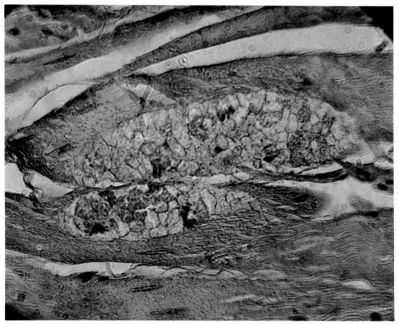

186. When an outbreak of *Plistophora mycotrophica* was observed in southern Europe, it was thought that this was a solitary occurrence of little general importance. However, a year later the same type of infection was found in two specimens of the rare New Zealand tuatara (*Sphenodon punctatum*) which had died in a New York zoo. The disease should be suspected whenever reptiles and amphibians which were well provided with food are found in an extreme state of cachexia. Photo: Elkan.

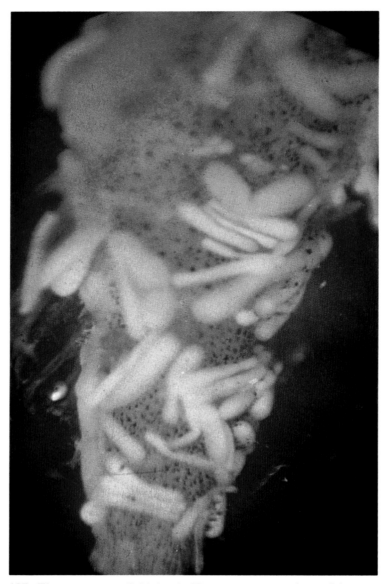

187. The common stickleback *(Gasterosteus aculeatus)* is occasionally found covered with elongated sausage-shaped, yellow-white cysts which are firmly embedded in the skin. Photo: Elkan.

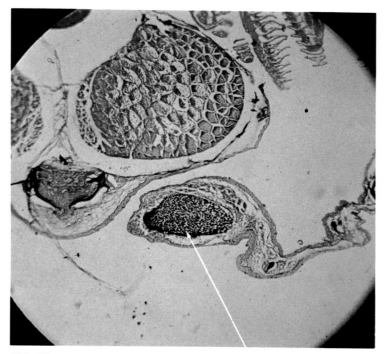

188. The cysts are filled with the developmental stages of a microsporidian *(Dermocystidium)* first observed in north German perch by Reichenbach-Klinke in 1950. Like the other microsporidians, *Dermocystidium* does not seem to interfere with the general health of the fish. Microsporidia occasionally also infest aquatic amphibia. There are many genera that are difficult to distinguish from one another. Photo: Elkan.

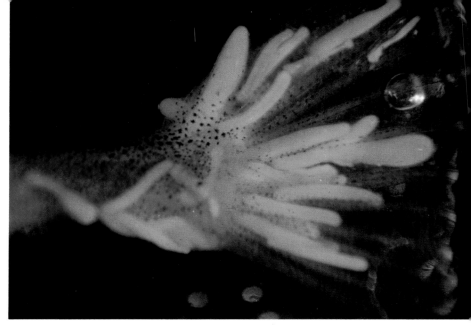

189. A first guide in the recognition of *Dermocystidium* is the shape of the cyst, which may be spherical, cylindrical or U-shaped. Photo: Elkan.

190. *Dermocystidium* sp. in the skin of *Paracheirodon innesi,* the neon tetra.

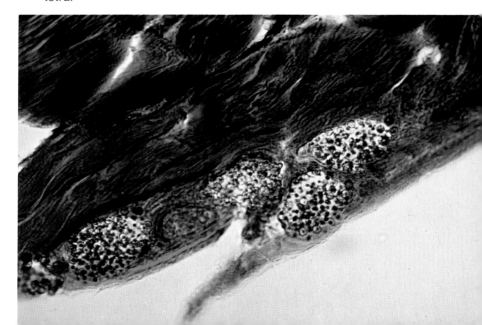

C. Monogenetic Trematodes

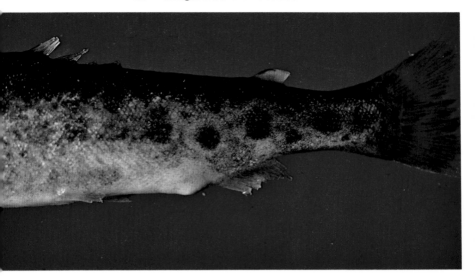

191. Fin necrosis due to gyrodactyliasis.

192. *Gyrodactylus* sp. feeding on the epithelial cells of fish skin.

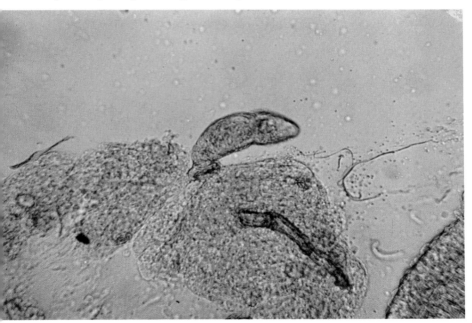

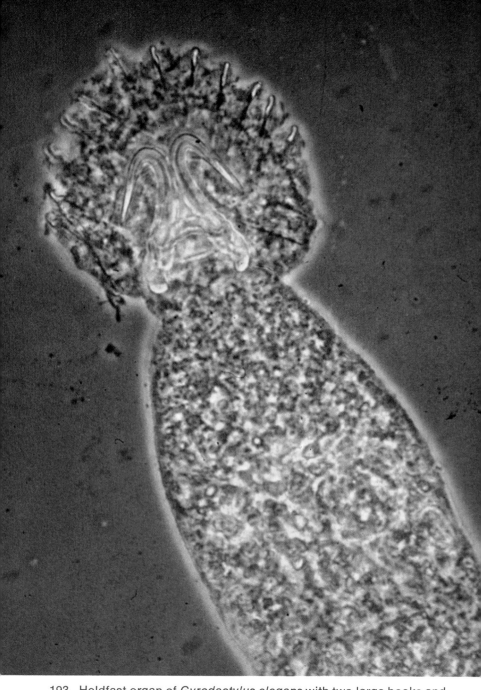

193. Holdfast organ of *Gyrodactylus elegans* with two large hooks and fourteen small hooklets. Photo: Frickhinger.

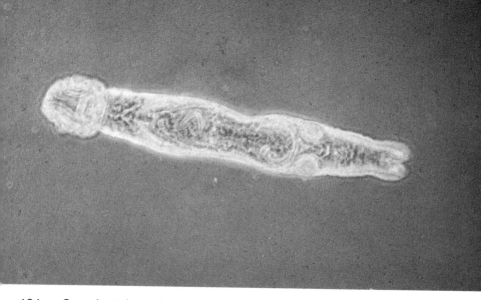

194.   *Gyrodactylus elegans*, a parasitic worm occurring on the gills and skin of fishes. The worms are supplied with rostral suckers and large caudal hooks. They are livebearing; note the young shown in the picture. Photo: Frickhinger.

195.   Eggs of *Dactylogyrus*. Note the elongated shape. The adults are parasitic on the gills of young fishes. Photo: Frickhinger.

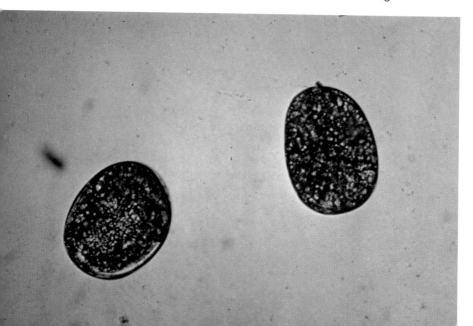

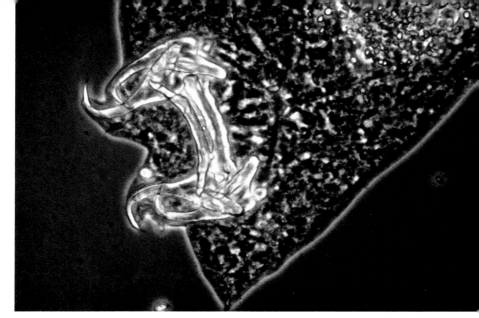

196. *Tetraonchus* sp. taken from a fish.

197. *Tetraonchus* sp., a trematode related to *Gyrodactylus*. The holdfast organ is supplied with four large hooks. Note the rostral suckers and the dark parts which represent yolk deposits. Photo: Frickhinger.

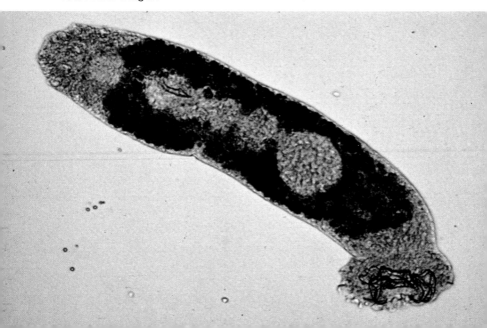

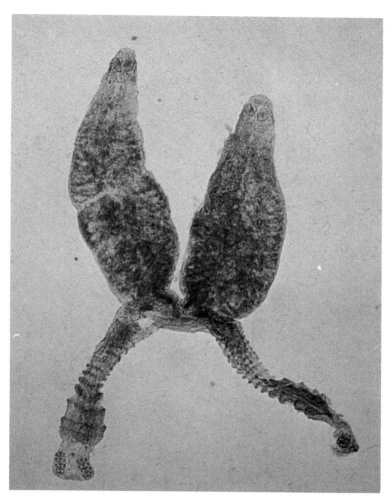

198. *Diplozoon nipponicum* from the gills of a goldfish *(Carassius auratus)*. These parasitic trematodes attach themselves to each other crosswise in pairs early in their development. They are hermaphrodites, each individual serving as male and female. They produce one egg each, filled with long filaments.

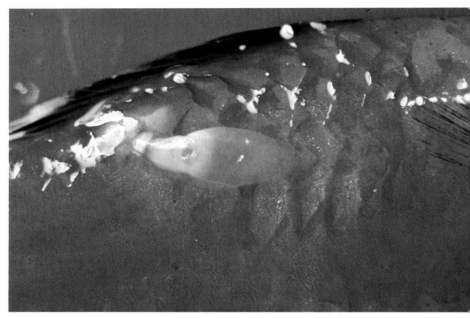

199. Monogenetic trematode attached to the skin of a fish.

200. Egg of *Microcotyle* sp. showing the typical long filaments.

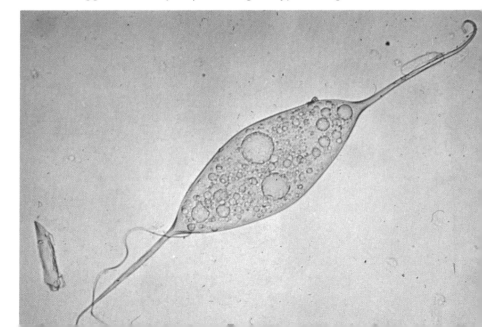

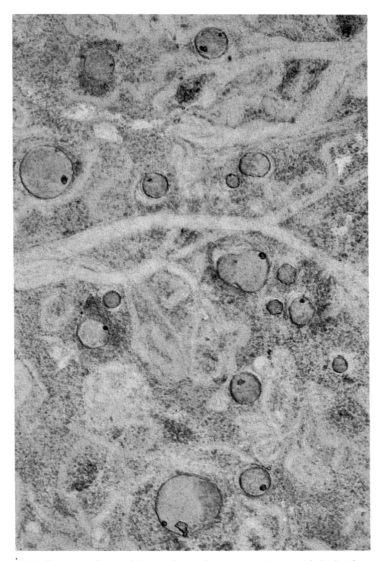

201. Eggs of *Sanguinicola inermis,* a trematode which, in the adult stage, lives in the blood of fish (blood worm). The worms may block the blood vessels, particularly those of the heart and the kidneys. The eggs are round or triangular with a blue spot. The first intermediate host is a snail.

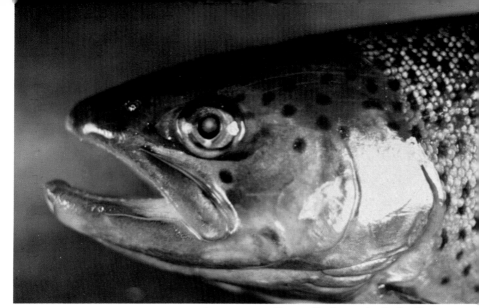

202. *Diplostomum spathaceum*, a digenetic trematode in the eye of a rainbow trout (*Salmo gairdneri*). The fish infects itself by feeding on parasitized snails which serve as second intermediate hosts. The final host is a fish-eating bird. The worms, which have an affinity for the eye, may cause blindness.

203. *Diplostomum spathaceum* taken from a fish. Isolated specimen with ventral haptor.

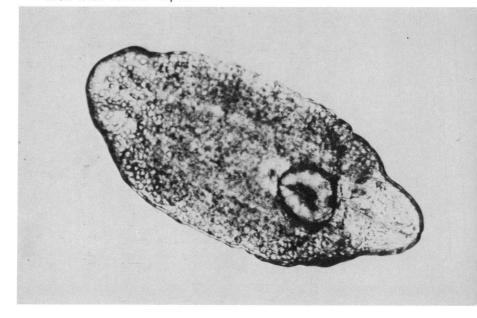

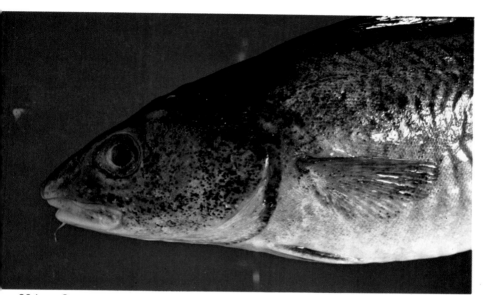

204.   *Cryptocotyle lingua* attached to the lower jaw of a cod.
205.   "Black spot" disease is caused by an assemblage of pigment cells around fluke metacercariae migrating through the skin from the gills.

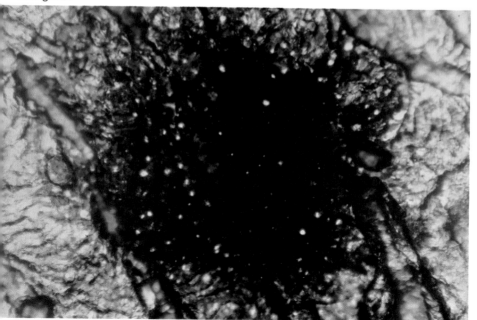

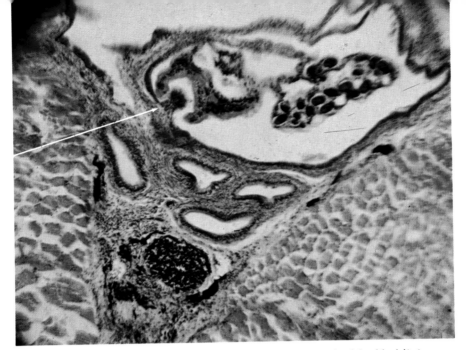

206. The stickleback (*Gasterosteus* sp.) seems to be the ideal habitat for fresh-water parasites. In the present case a flat worm can be seen attached to the wall of the bladder of the fish. Note, on the left, the oral sucker of the worm attached to a small fold in the mucous lining of the bladder. The right part of the worm contains developing eggs. Photo: Elkan.

207. *Syncoelium* sp., a digenetic trematode with branched ventral sucker from *Eques* sp. Photo: Frickhinger.

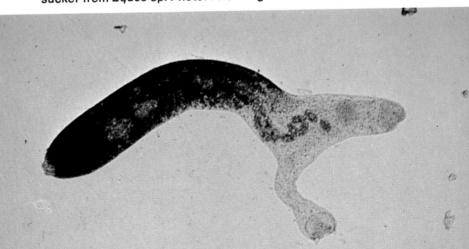

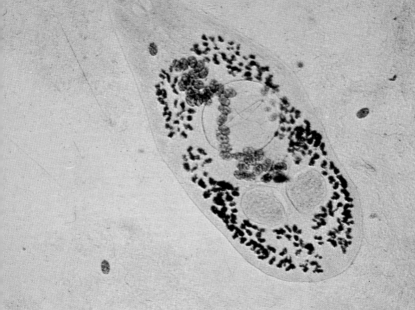

208.   A digenetic trematode from the intestine of a fish. These worms are equipped with a rostral and ventral sucker but have no hooks. Most of them need two intermediate hosts to complete their development. The majority of these intermediate hosts are snails or clams. Photo: Frickhinger.

209.   A larval digenetic trematode taken from a cyst under the skin of *Amblydoras* sp. Photo: Frickhinger.

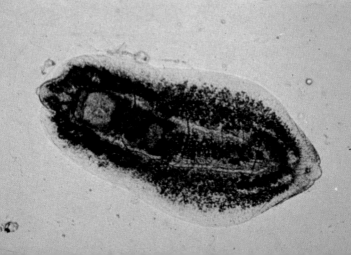

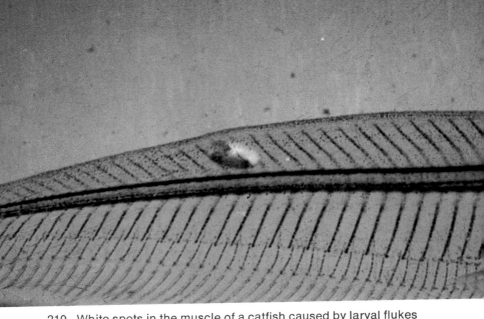

210. White spots in the muscle of a catfish caused by larval flukes (metacercariae). Photo: Frickhinger.

211. A cyst containing a larval fluke from the liver of a cichlid. Photo: Frickhinger.

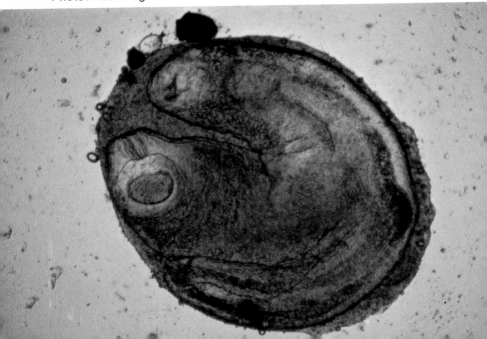

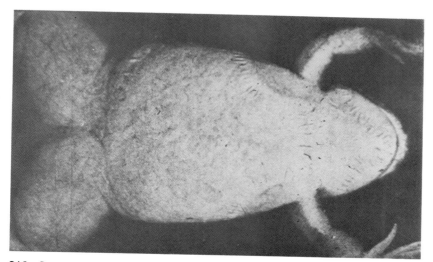

212. Some trematodes may invade aquatic frogs by penetrating their skin at a period in their development when the larvae (cercariae) swim freely in the water. They seem unable to penetrate the intact skin but may gain entrance through areas supplied with sensory nerve endings (neuromasts). This photograph shows how these neuromasts are arranged like stitches in the skin of *Xenopus laevis*. In the healthy frog the neuromasts are distinguishable as white marks on the dark skin. Photo: Elkan.

213. In an infected frog the relation is reversed. All the neuromasts are black against a pale skin. Photo: Elkan.

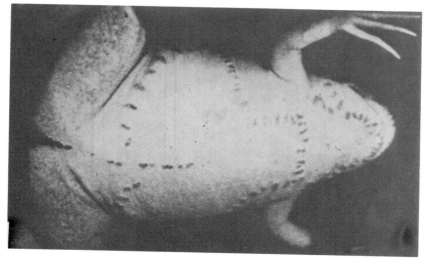

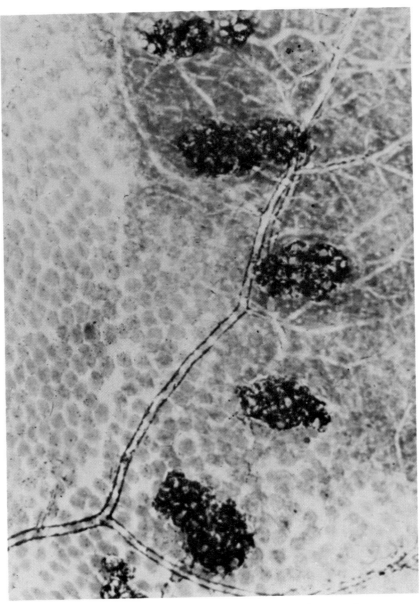

214. The reason for the neuromast color change can be seen by looking at the underside of the skin. Under each neuromast are a number of cysts and an accumulation of black pigment-carrying cells (melanocytes). Photo: Elkan.

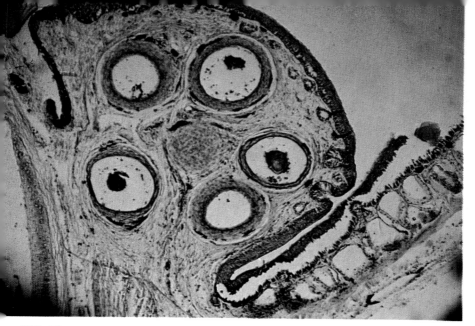

215. The true nature of the condition appears in a section through the affected skin. The parasites (strigeid cercariae) have penetrated the skin and encysted. Photo: Elkan.

216. Each cyst contains one larva. They remain in this state until the frog is eaten by a predator (birds of prey, small mammals, crocodiles, etc.). Then the capsule is digested, the larva liberated and freed to develop toward its mature stage. Photo: Elkan.

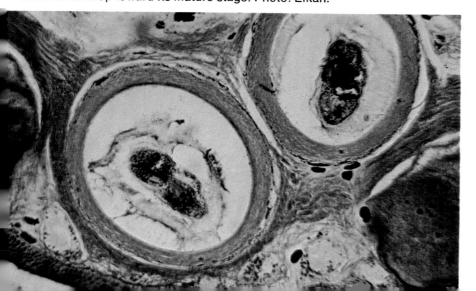

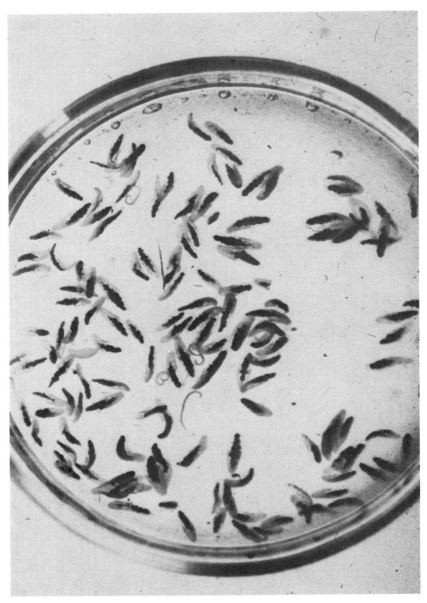

217. *Ochetosoma grandispinus* is a small trematode which inhabits the intestinal canal of North American snakes. The specimens shown came from the mouth and esophagus of *Drymarchon corais couperi*. Photo: Elkan.

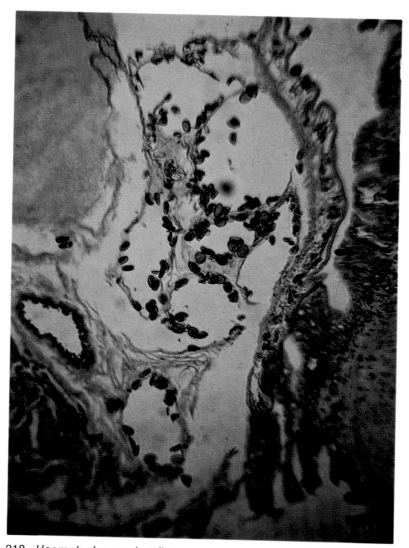

218. *Haemolychus* sp. is a flatworm commonly found in the lungs of frogs, where it thrives on cellular debris and the frog's blood cells. In section we see either the worm or its eggs. Photo: Elkan.

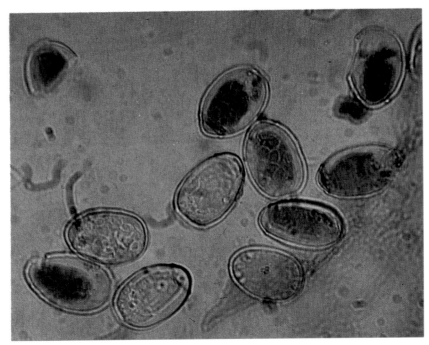

219. The eggs of *Haemolychus* sp. are provided with a 'lid' which opens when the embryo emerges. Photo: Elkan.

220. *Macrodera longicollis* is a common pulmonary parasite of snakes. Photo: Elkan.

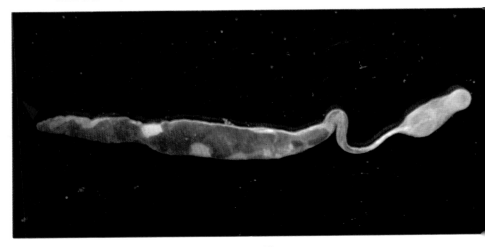

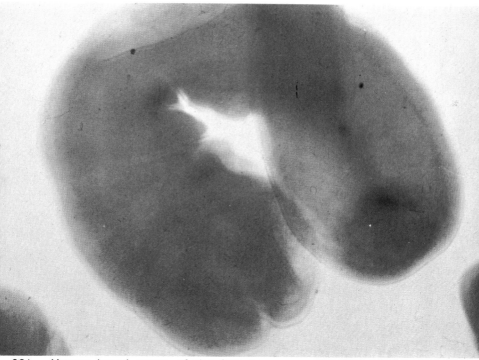

221.   Young larval stage of the fish tapeworm *Diphyllobothrium* sp., armed with the sucker typical of the species. A copepod serves as first host, and man can be the final host. Photo: Reichenbach-Klinke.

222.   Section through a cyst containing a larva of *Diphyllobothrium* sp. Photo: Reichenbach-Klinke.

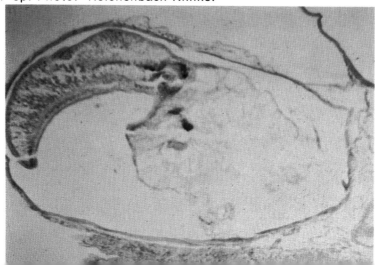

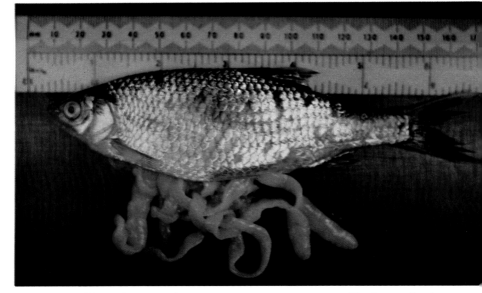

223. *Ligula intestinalis* in the body cavity of a roach *(Rutilus rutilus)*.

224. The larval form of *Ligula intestinalis* can reach the length of one meter and is found in the body cavity of fish, compressing and damaging the intestinal organs and causing sterility. The final host is a fish-eating bird. The picture shows the dissection of a fish infected with *Ligula intestinalis*.

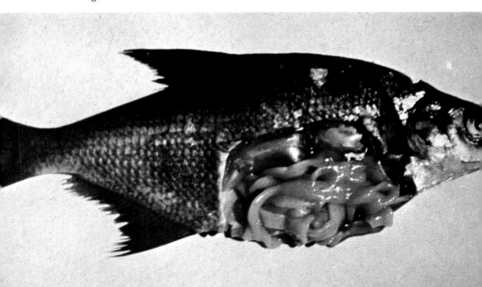

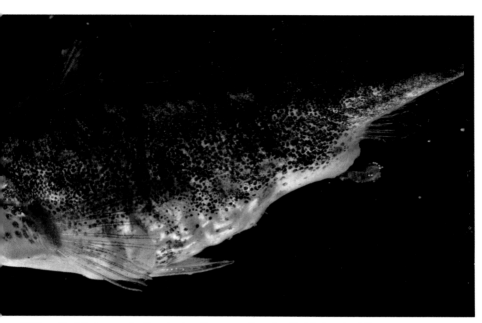

225. Schistocephaliasis in three-spined stickleback (*Gasterosteus aculeatus*).

226. Sagittal section through a stickleback (*Gasterosteus aculeatus*). The tapeworm *Schistocephalus solidus* infects the stickleback while in a larval (plerocercoid) form and grows to such a size that it displaces the intestines of the fish. Photo: Elkan.

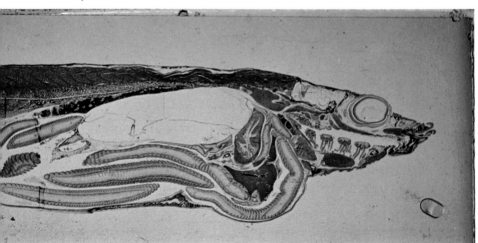

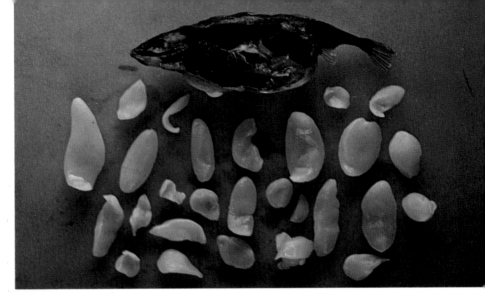

227. Stickleback *(Gasterosteus aculeatus)* infected with *Schisto-cephalus solidus* and *Glugea anomala.* Little remains of the normal anatomy of the fish. Photo: Elkan.

228. In Israel, where *Tilapia zilli* is extensively bred for the table, it has been observed that one-eyed blindness occasionally occurs in these fish. The cause of this deficiency can be seen in this picture. The plerocercoid larva of a tapeworm encysts itself immediately behind the eyeball, adjacent to the optic nerve. The pressure exerted by the cyst puts the eye out of action. Photo: Elkan.

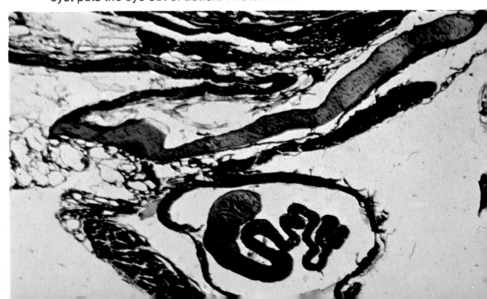

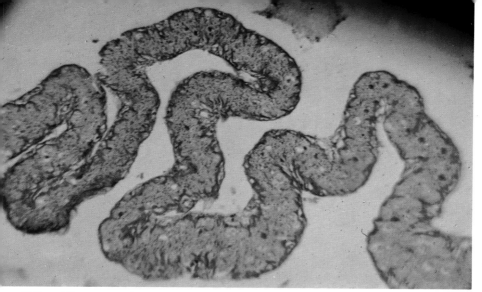

229. Close-up of part of the pleorcercoid shown in figure 228.

230. The muscle of a whitefish (*Coregonus lavaretus*) dissected to show the presence of larvae of the tapeworm *Triaenophorus crassus*. One cyst has been opened. Photo: Zool. -Par. Inst. Munich.

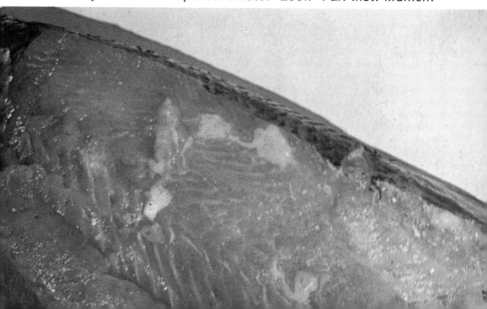

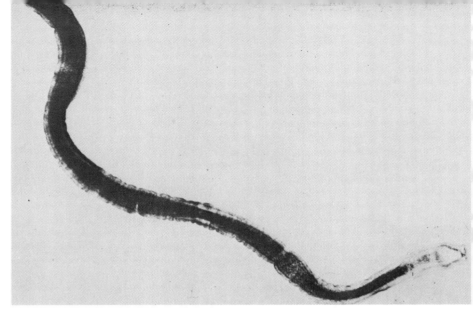

231. Juvenile *Triaenophorus nodulosus* taken from a fish.

232. Scolex of *Triaenophorus crassus* showing the four hooks typical of the species. The worms are harmless to humans because they are digested in the stomach, but affected fish are difficult to sell because of the poor appearance of the tissue.

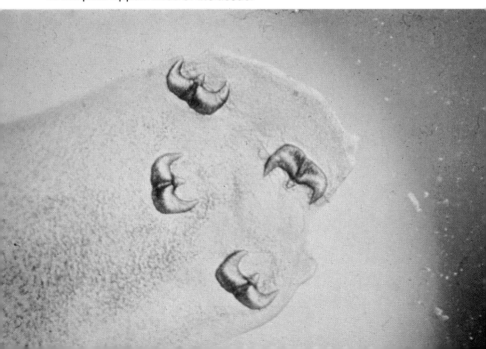

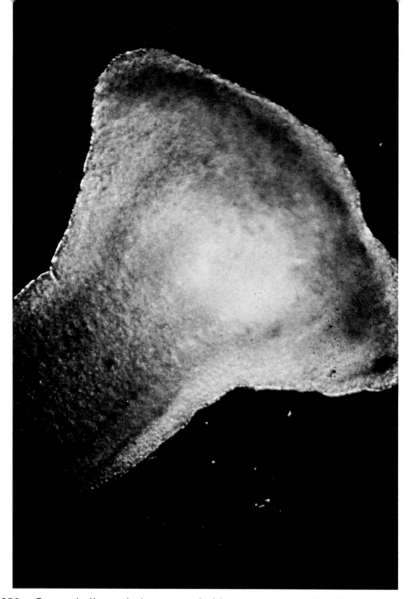

233. *Caryophyllaeus laticeps,* a primitive tapeworm with only one proglottid containing the single testis and ovary. The picture shows the rostral end of the worm, which has no typical holdfast organ but which can expand to assume the shape of a flower (caryophyllid). The parasite occurs in juvenile carp and in other cyprinid fish. The life cycle starts with the entry into the first intermediate host, a segmented worm of the genera *Tubifex* or *Limnodrilus.*

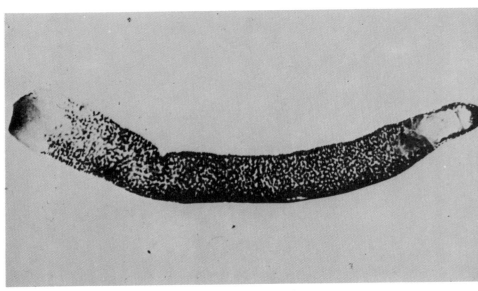

234. *Caryophyllaeides fennica* taken from a bream.

235. *Proteocephalus pillicollis* taken from a three-spined stickleback (*Gasterosteus aculeatus*).

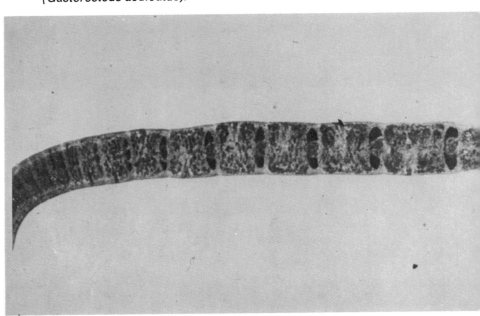

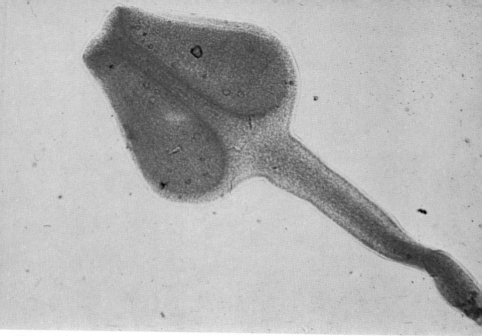

236. Scolex of *Bothriocephalus* sp., an intestinal tapeworm of cyprinid fishes, armed with four suckers.

237. *Proteocephalus (Ichthyotaenia)* sp., a tapeworm whose scolex is armed with five suckers. The worms abound in the intestines of many fishes. The first intermediate hosts are water fleas (copepods). The picture shows several proglottids with maturing eggs.

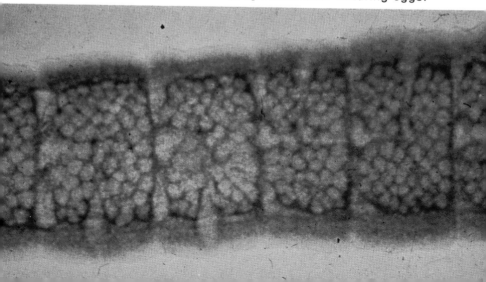

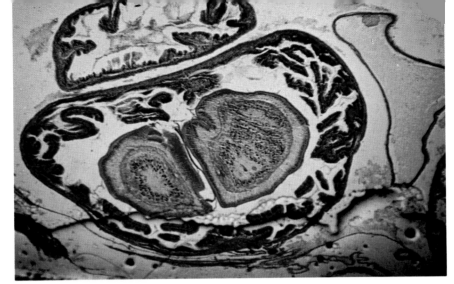

238. The picture shows a transverse section through a tapeworm
found in the intestine of a New Guinea frog *(Nyctimistes daymani)*.
Although a tapeworm of this size will certainly interfere with the host's
metabolism, it will, in most cases, not kill it unless it becomes large or
numerous enough to cause intestinal obstruction. Photo: Elkan.

239. *Cephalochlamys namaquensis* is a small tapeworm which is
found in about 7% of all *Xenopus laevis* frogs imported from South
Africa. When, in the course of being used for pregnancy tests, the frogs
were once injected with an extract containing small amounts of
bromphenol, the worms were expelled. The picture shows two fully
grown specimens of the worm. Photo: Elkan.

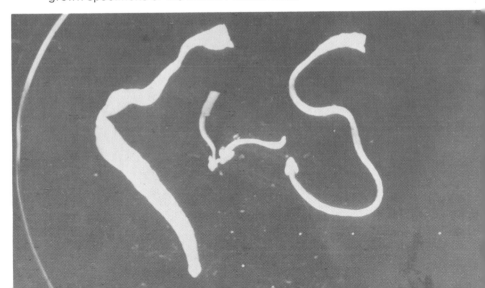

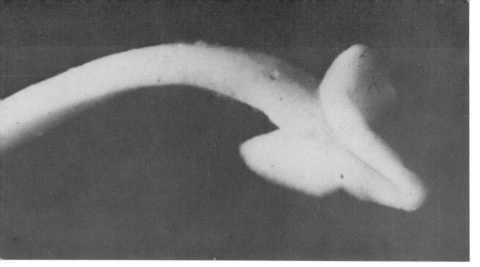

240. The holdfast organ of *Cephalochlamys namaquensis* has two lateral grooves which can be used to fix the worm to the intestinal mucosa of the host. Photo: Elkan.

241. The picture shows a section through the holdfast organ of *Cephalochlamys namaquensis* attached to the intestinal wall. The worm invaginates but does not penetrate the mucosa. No obvious defence reaction on the part of the host can be seen. Photo: Elkan.

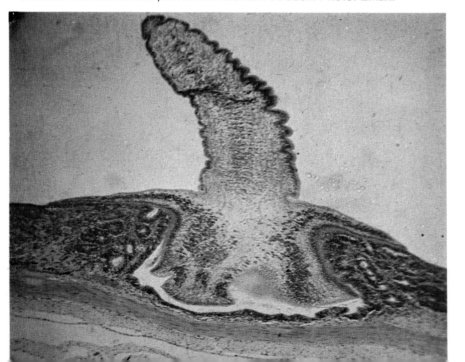

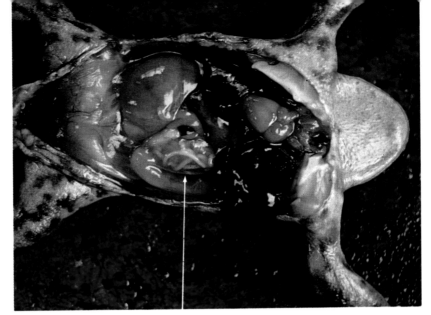

242. *Nematotaenia* sp. is a small cestode which is found in almost every specimen of the common European grass frog *(Rana temporaria)* examined. It is not at all unusual for this worm to occur in such numbers that it completely blocks the intestinal canal, causing the death of the frog. The picture shows a case of this kind. The worms can plainly be seen through the thinned out wall of the intestine. The frog died of intestinal obstruction. Photo: Elkan.

243. The scolex of *Nematotaenia dispar*. The holdfast organ of this worm looks very much like that of other cestodes. It is armed with four suckers. Photo: Elkan.

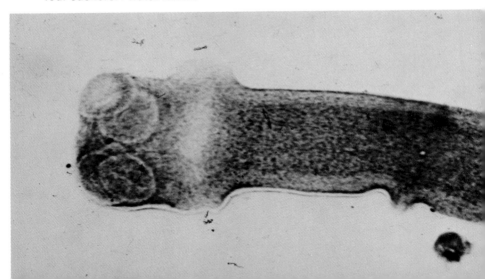

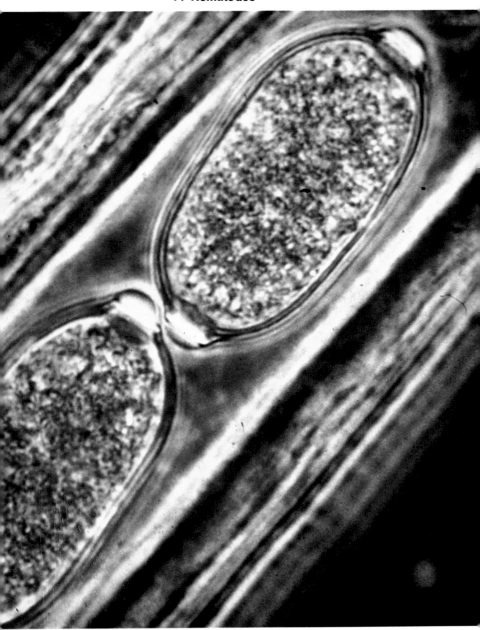

244. Eggs of the hair worm (*Capillaria* sp.), a worm found in the gut or in the liver of fish. Photo: Frickhinger.

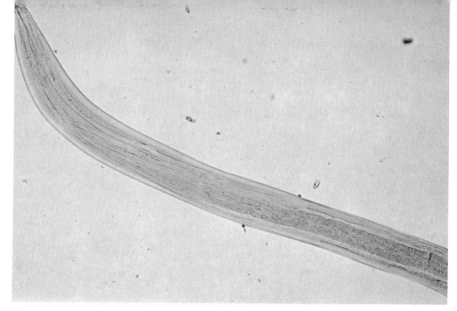

245. The larval stage of *Contracaecum aduncum*, a nematode in the gastrointestinal canal and rarely in the muscular tissue of fish. The first intermediate host is a copepod.

246. *Cystidicola* sp. in the swim bladder of a rainbow trout *(Salmo gairdneri)*.

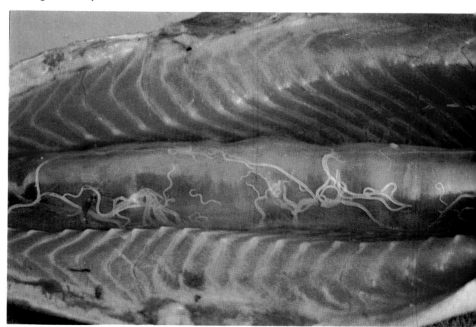

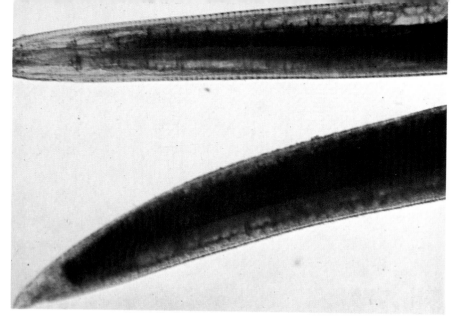

247. *Philometra (Thwaitia) abdominalis,* the blood worm, lives under the gill cover or in the body cavity of fish. The intermediate host of this worm is a copepod.

248. Microfilaria of *Philometra* sp. in the blood of an eel *(Anguilla anguilla).*

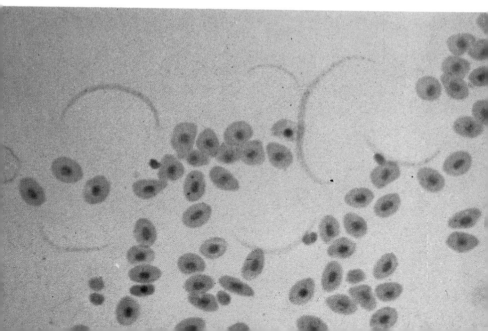

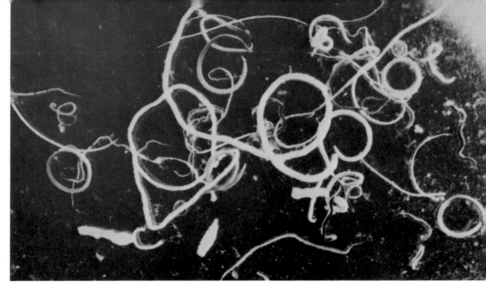

249. Just as in the case of the flat worms, the number of round worms we may find in any one animal is sometimes considerable. The picture shows a collection of worms made from the intestine of a single European common toad *(Bufo bufo)*. Most of the worms are round worms, but a few acanthocephalans are also present. Photo: Elkan.

250. The photograph shows a collection of round worms *(Polydelphis oculata)* obtained from one specimen of *Python reticulatus.* Photo: Elkan.

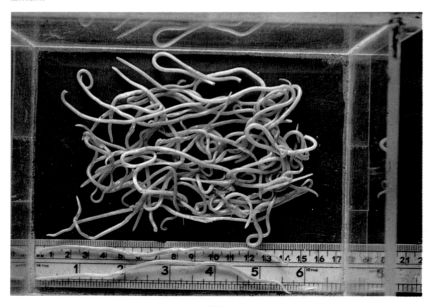

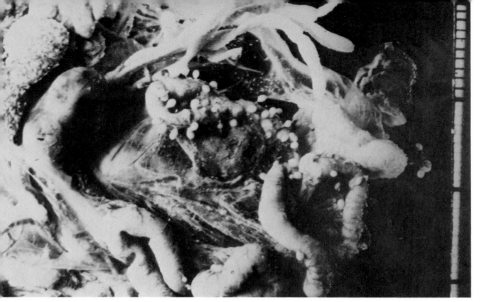

251. Nematodes do not always complete their development in one host. A group of Surinam water toads *(Pipa pipa)* was found heavily infected by nematode larvae encysted in the peritoneum. Photo: Elkan.

252. Nematode cysts found in the muscles of the frog *Rana occipitalis.* Photo: Elkan.

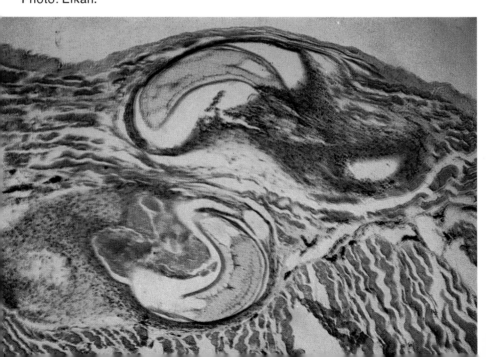

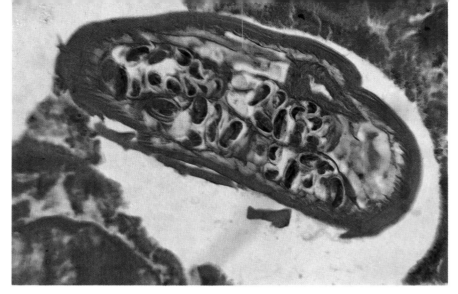

253. The picture shows a longitudinal section through a nematode found in the intestine of an Australian water skink *(Sphenomorphus quoyi)*. The embryos in the worm's eggs are seen in the early stages of development. Photo: Elkan.

254. Transverse section of a nematode found in the intestinal canal of *Sphenomorphus quoyi*. The embryos are in an advanced stage of development. Photo: Elkan.

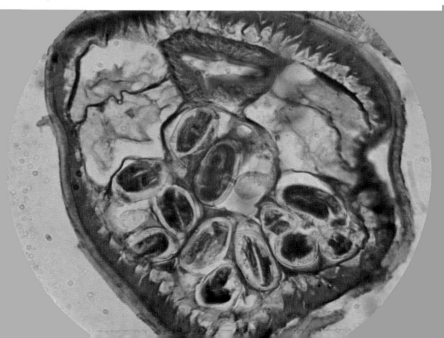

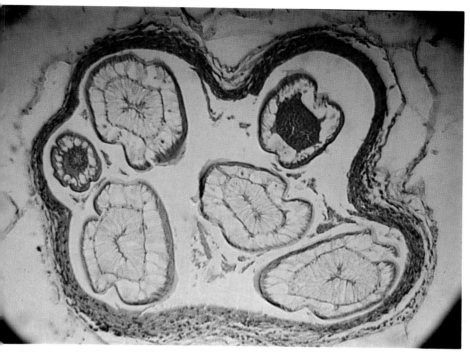

255. In a specimen of *Rana occipitalis,* sections of the intestine revealed the presence of nematodes. It is not possible to determine from sections alone the exact species of worm encountered, but the differences in their general anatomy allow at least differentiation between the five main groups of helminths. Phóto: Elkan.

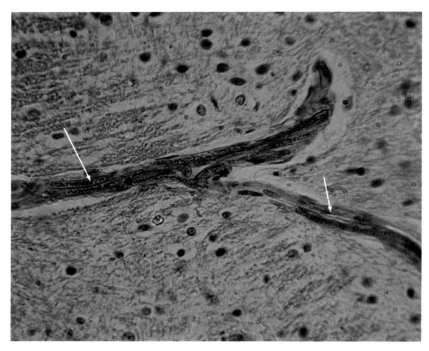

256. *Physignathus leseuri,* the Australian water dragon, infected with *Capillaria* sp. These round worms are so small that they can be carried about in the host's blood stream. They cannot be seen with the naked eye. By obstructing small capillaries they can cause considerable damage and even death. In the case presented here, the lizard had been in captivity for seven years before it died from unknown causes. The picture shows *Capillaria* sp. obstructing small blood vessels in the brain. Similar pictures were obtained from every other organ. Since the lizard could not have become infected in England, the infection must have taken at least seven years to develop. Photo: Elkan.

G. Acanthocephalans

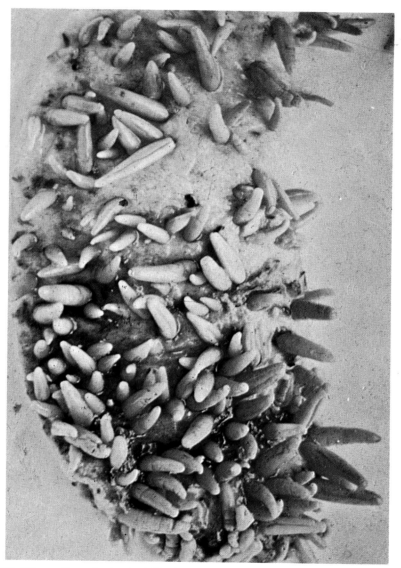

257. Dissection of a barbel *(Barbus barbus)* with several specimens of the acanthocephalan *Pomphorhynchus laevis*. The Acanthocephala are armed with a proboscis which is covered with rows of small hooks. The proboscis, which is retractile, can penetrate the intestinal wall of the host. The body of the worm remains floating in the intestinal lumen. Food intake occurs by osmosis.

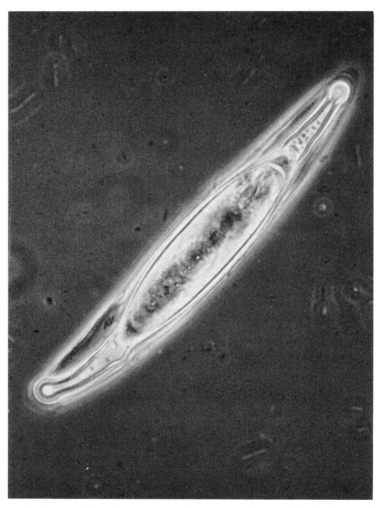

258. Eggs of *Pomphorhynchus laevis* show the hooks of the larval worm (acanthella). Large numbers of these eggs may be found in the intestinal canal. Photo: Frickhinger.

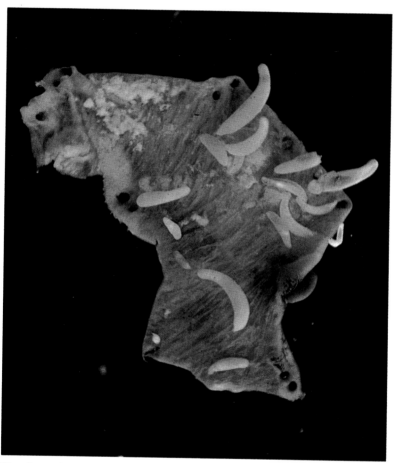

259. Acanthocephalans, commonly known as thorny-headed worms, parasitize mammals and birds as well as lower vertebrates. The organ on which they carry their formidable array of spines or barbed hooks is not the head but a proboscis, a prolongation of the body which buries itself deep in the wall of the host's intestine. The picture shows several *Acanthocephalus ranae* firmly attached to the gastric lining of a common toad (*Bufo bufo*). These worms have no digestive canal. Once attached to the host, they absorb nutritive matter through their surface, and they cannot later detach themselves. Photo: Elkan.

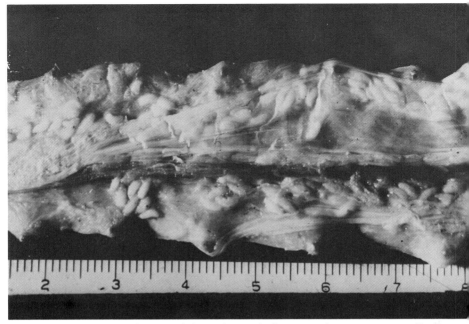

260. The larval forms of Acanthocephalans are known as acanthella. Shown encysted in large numbers under the peritoneum of an indigo snake (*Drymarchon corais couperi*) are acanthella of *Acanthocephalus* sp. Photo: Elkan.

261. The proboscis of *Acanthocephalus ranae*. Photo: Elkan.

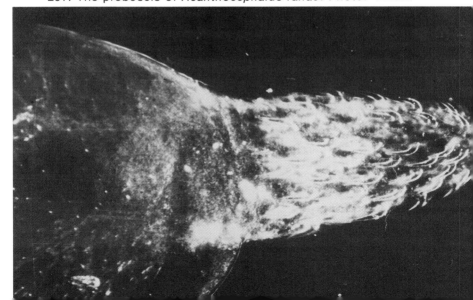

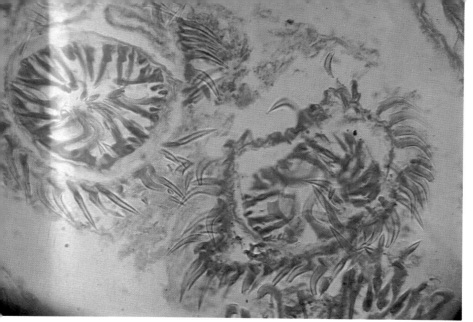

262. The spines covering the holdfast organ of acanthocephalans are particularly well visible in dark field illumination. The picture shows an acanthella from the intestine of an Australian lizard *(Lialis burtoni)*. Photo: Elkan.

263. Dark field illumination of an acanthella taken from the intestine of an Australian lizard *(Lialis burtoni)*. Photo: Elkan.

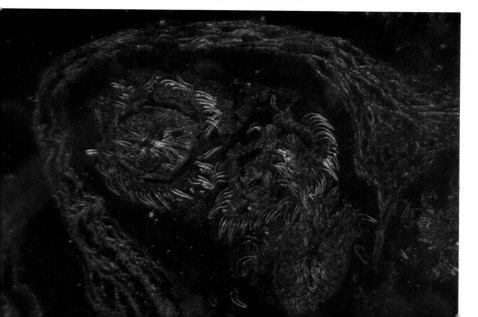

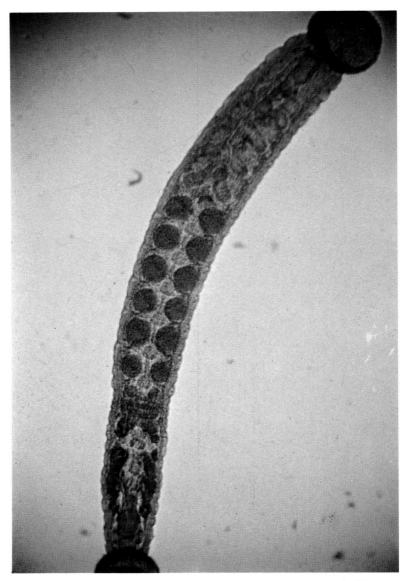

264. *Hemiclepsis marginata,* the European broad fish leech. Photo: Zool.-Parasit. Inst. Munich.

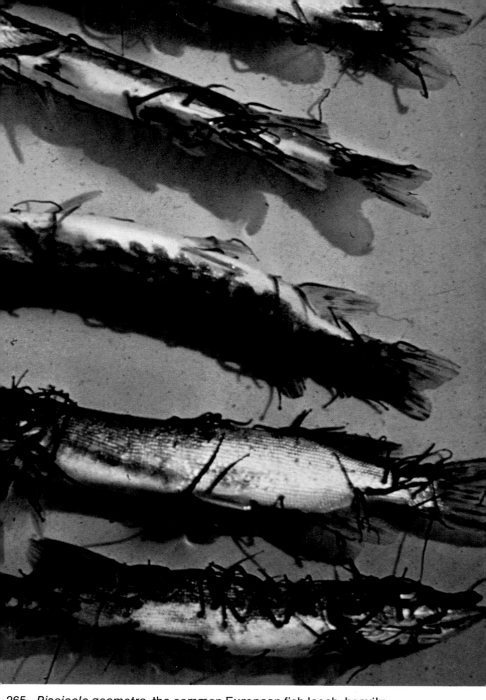

265. *Piscicola geometra,* the common European fish leech, heavily infesting juvenile pike (*Esox* sp.). Photo: Bayr. Biol. Versuchsanstalt.

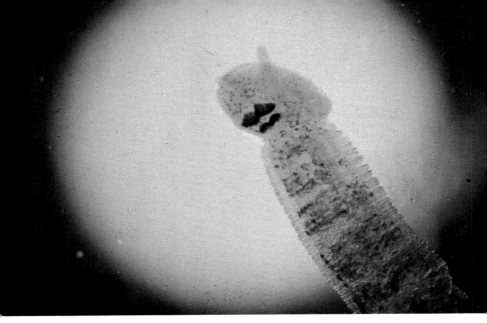

266. Oral sucker of *Piscicola geometra.* Note the crescent-shaped eyes.

267. *Branchiobdella parasita,* a segmented worm which parasitizes crayfish. The picture shows the anterior part of the worm with the black teeth, and the caudal part with the sucker.

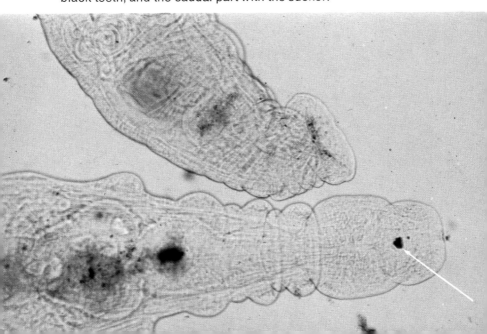

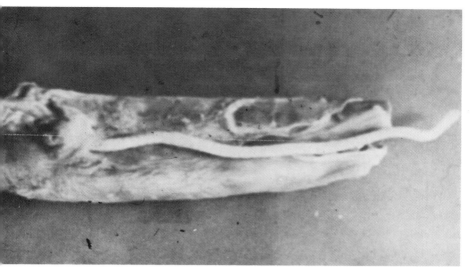

268. The picture shows *Kiricephalus coarctatus* in the stomach wall of a North American snake; the worm-like animal, which despite its appearance is more closely related to the spiders than to the worms, had burrowed through the wall into the adjoining liver, which had become adherent to the stomach. The body of the parasite was lying free in the snake's stomach. *Kiricephalus* and its relatives are not often seen in the lower vertebrates of the Northern Hemisphere, but they are quite common in some areas of the tropics. The holdfast organ is armed with four hooks, and the body is segmented; there is a mouth, an intestinal canal and an anus. Photo: Elkan.

269. *Kiricephalus coarctatus* dissected from the stomach of a snake. Photo: Elkan.

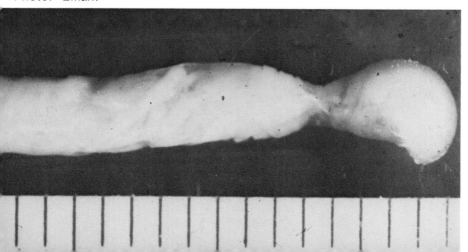

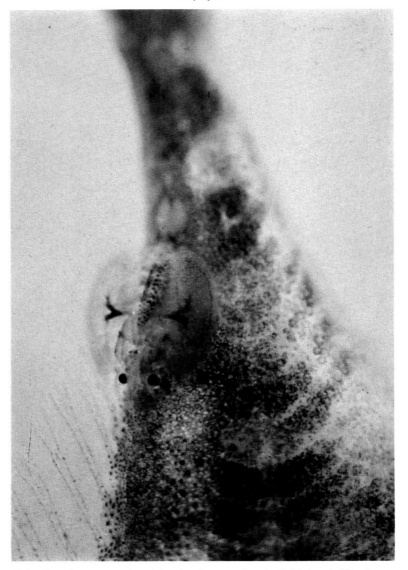

270. *Argulus* sp. on the skin of a three-spined stickleback *(Gasterosteus aculeatus).*

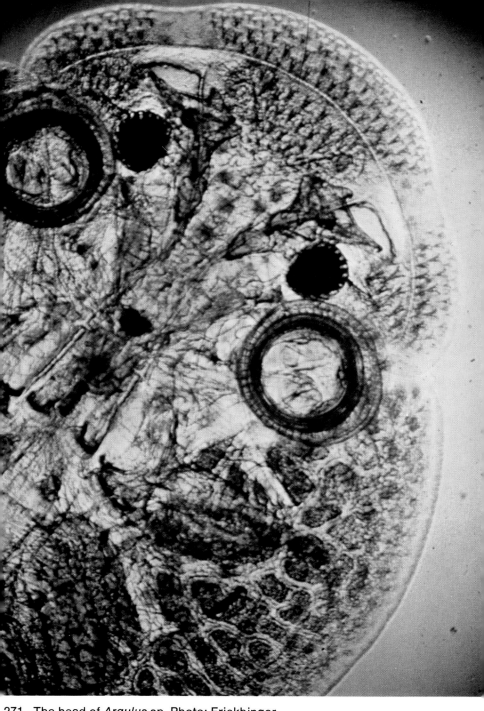

271. The head of *Argulus* sp. Photo: Frickhinger.

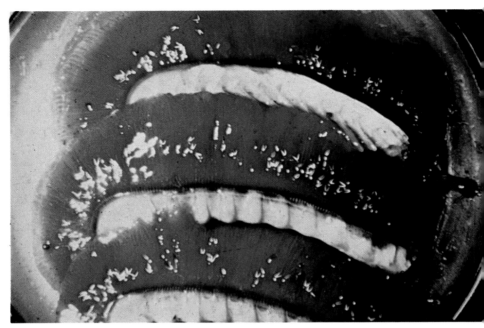

272. *Ergasilus* sp. on the gills of a bream. Photo: Dr. P. de Kinkelin.

273. *Ergasilus sieboldi*, the common gill copepod of fish. The female is recognized by the presence of egg sacs. Note the prehensile antennae and the single eye.

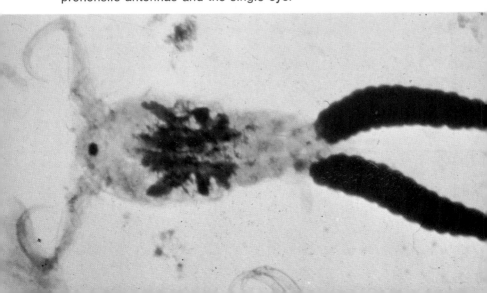

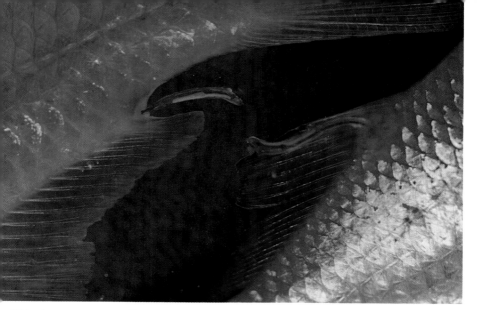

274. *Lernaea carassii,* a copepod parasitizing the skin of goldfish *(Carassius auratus).* Photo: Frickhinger.

275. Head of *Lernaea* sp. showing the attaching mechanism. Photo: Frickhinger.

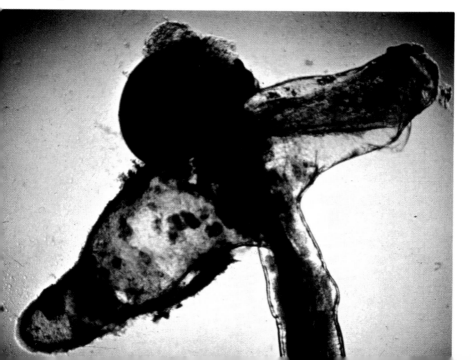

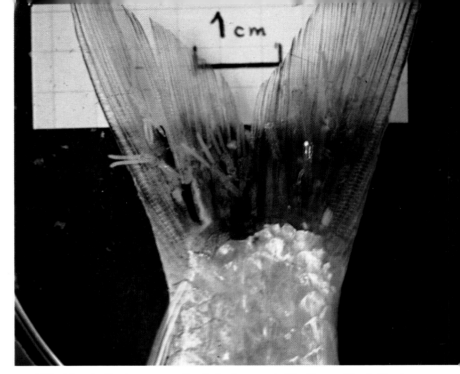

276. *Tracheliastes* sp. on the tail of a roach *(Rutilus rutilus)*. Photo:
Dr. P. de Kinkelin.

277. *Anchistratos* sp., a parasitic copepod on the gills of a trunk fish
(Ostracion cyanurus). Photo: Frickhinger.

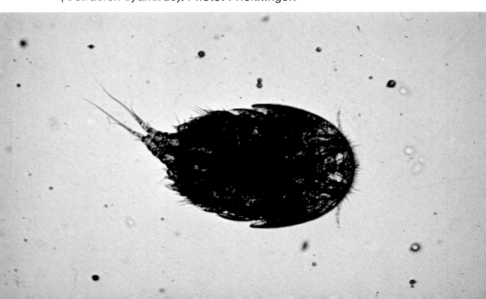

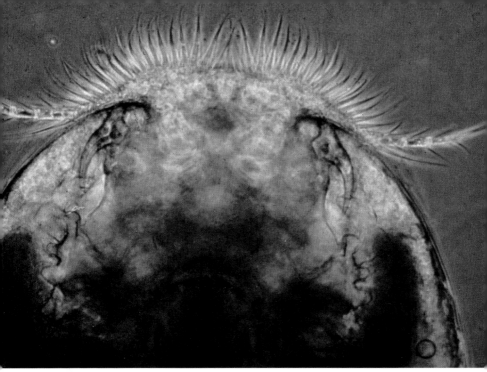

278. Head of the copepod shown in figure 277. Note the single red eye and the feathery antenna. Photo: Frickhinger.

279. *Lepeophtheirus salmonis* taken from a salmonid fish.

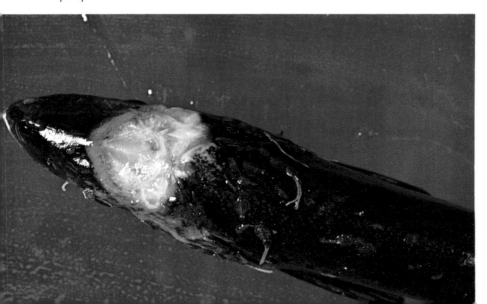

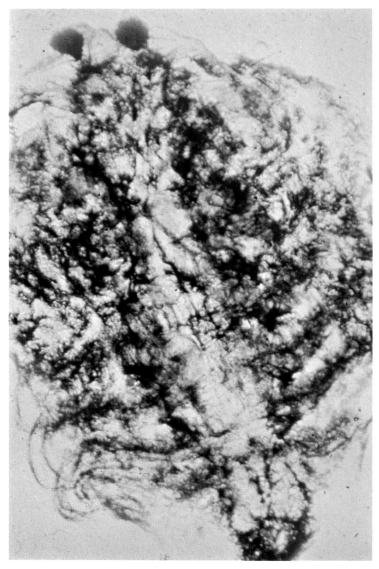

280. *Dolops* sp., a South American copepod parasitizing the skin of various fish.

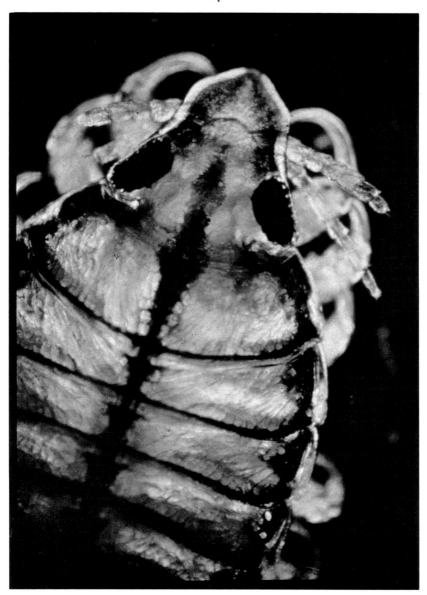

281. An isopod parasitizing fish. These South American parasites attach themselves to the skin, which they pierce by means of a stylet. They live by sucking blood and fluid from the body of the fish. Note the hooked appendages and the large eyes. Photo: Frickhinger.

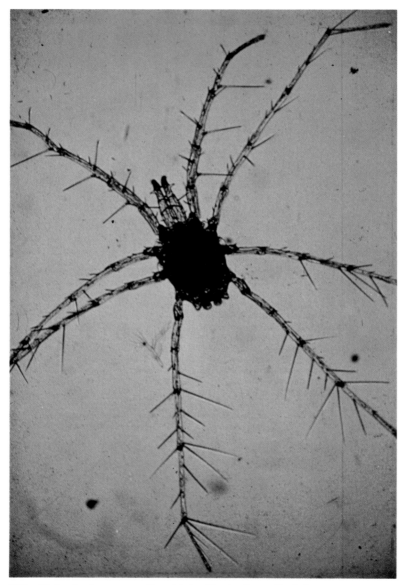

282. *Unionicola* sp., a mite which attacks juvenile fish.

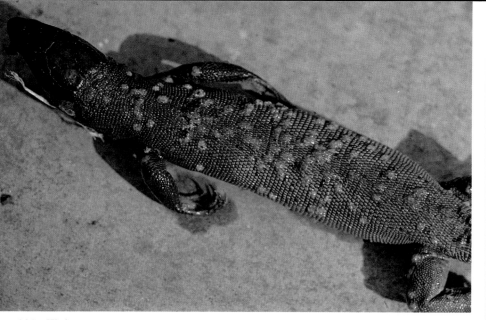

283. Ticks may attack and occasionally even kill small vertebrates. The picture shows a European green lizard *(Lacerta viridis)* attacked by ticks. The ticks attach themselves to the skin of the host, pierce it with their proboscis and feed by sucking blood from the dermal capillaries. To keep the wound open they secrete substances which prevent it from healing. In some cases this chronic irritation causes the skin to produce warty growths. The tick will be found buried in these. Photo: Elkan.

284. *Amblyomma sparsum* attached to a black mamba *(Dendraspis jamesi).* Photo: Elkan.

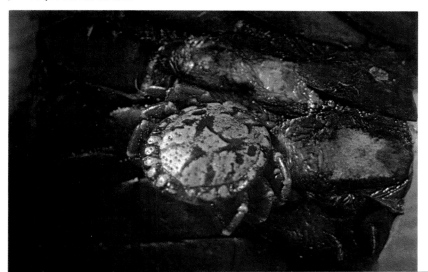

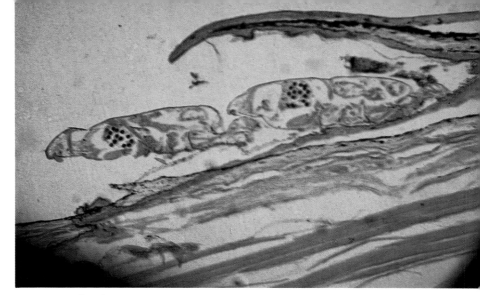

285. *Ophionyssus natricis,* the common snake mite. Two individuals are here seen lying head to tail under one of the scales of a garter snake *(Thamnophis sirtalis).* Photo: Elkan.

286. The proboscis of *Ophionyssus natricis.* Ticks are known to transmit viral and bacterial diseases. In this picture the tick can be seen dipping into a pool of bacteria. (Gram-Weigert stain). Photo: Elkan.

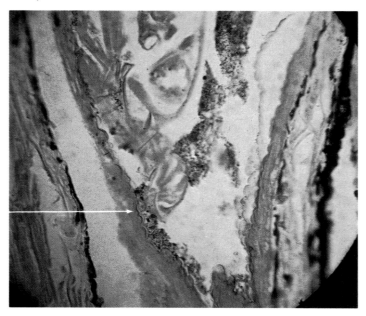

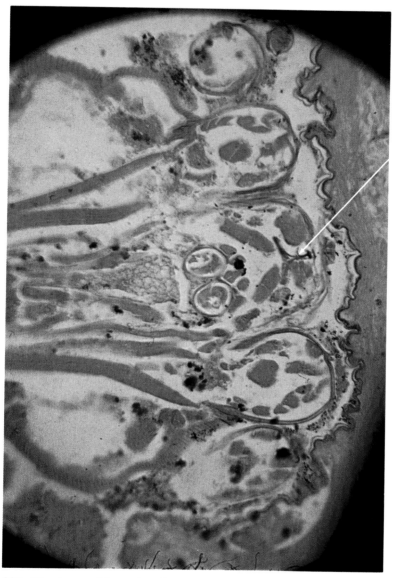

287. The brown triangular structure is the pharyngeal pump of *Ophionyssus natricis* which conveys blood and serum from the victim to the parasite. Photo: Elkan.

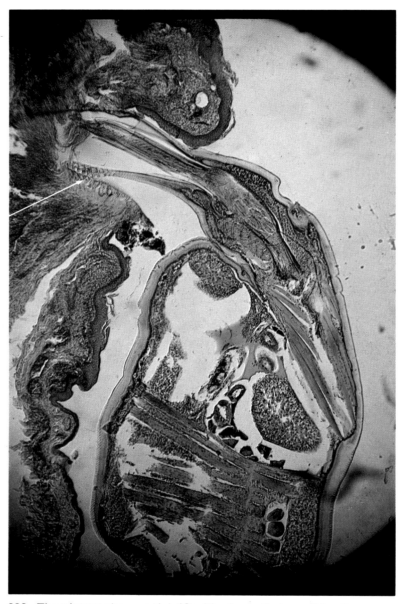

288. The picture shows a tick *(Ornithodorus tholuzani)* feeding on a rat. The picture would not look different if the victim were a snake or lizard. Note the saw-like edges of the hypostome cutting through the skin of the victim. Photo: Elkan.

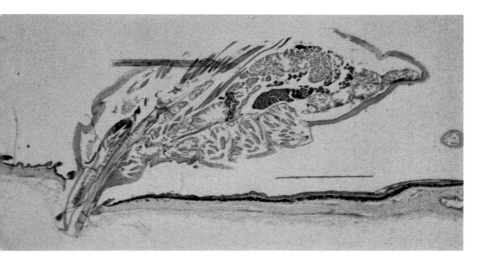

289. *Amblyomma sparsum* parasitizing the skin of a black mamba *(Dendraspis jamesi)*. Photo: Elkan.

290. *Amblyomma sparsum* cutting through the skin of a black mamba *(Dendraspis jamesi)*. Note the yellow substance which glues together the layers of the snake's skin and forms a tube through which the tick's proboscis can move. Photo: Elkan.

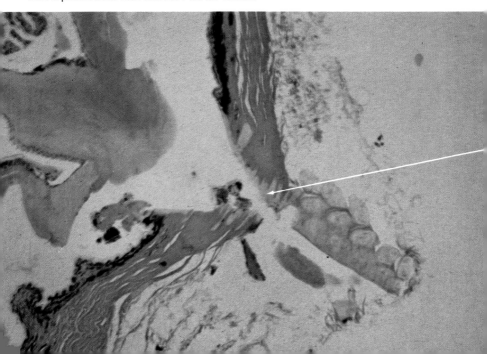

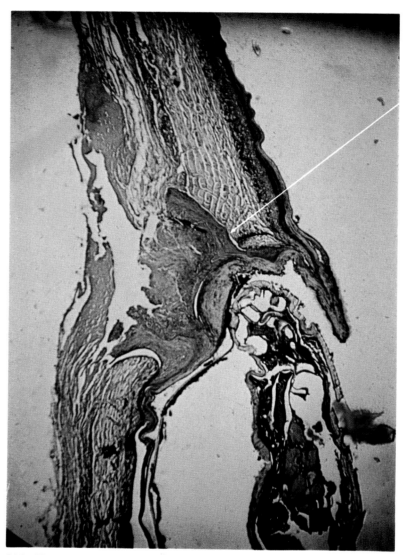

291. Ticks are attracted to areas on the victim's skin where there may already be a break of the skin caused by accident, inflammation or ulceration. In the picture the tick has not pierced the skin and indeed it had no need to do so because there was in existence a small ulcer which had already destroyed the layers of the skin down to the subcutis. All the tick had to do was to feed on the secretion from the ulcer. Note the sharply interrupted fibers of the *stratum compactum* of the dermis. Photo: Elkan.

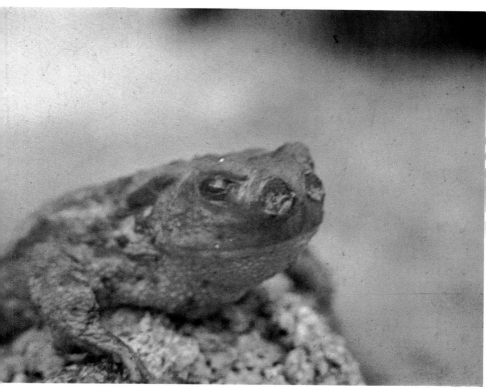

292. Some genera of flies, both in Europe and in tropical countries, particularly in Australia, have learned to lay their eggs on the hind legs of frogs. The maggots, when hatched, creep forward and gain access to the frog's tissue via the eyes or the nose. They begin at once to feed on the frog's substance. The picture shows *Lucilia bufonivora* feeding on a common toad *(Bufo bufo)*. The toad, which apparently has no defence against this invasion, soon dies and thereby provides further food for the voracious maggots. Photo: Elkan.

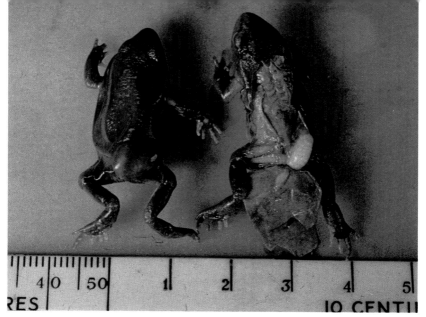

293. An Australian toad *(Pseudophryne bibroni)* attacked by two maggots of a fly *(Batrachomyia* sp.) which have gained access to the dorsal lymph sac. Photo: Elkan.

294. One of the *Batrachomyia* sp. maggots has pierced the body wall and inserted its feeding parts into the body cavity of the toad, where it can be seen lying among the intestines. The maggots leave the toad when they are ready to pupate. It is not recorded what happens to the toad. Photo: Elkan.

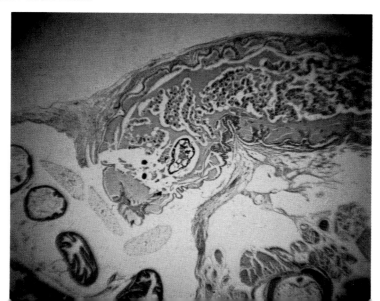

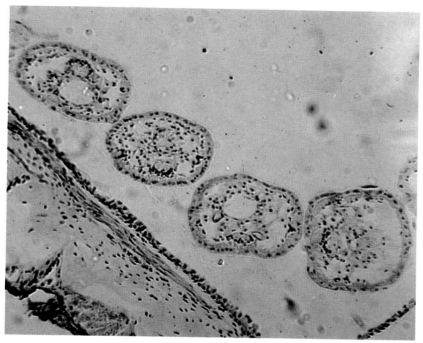

295. Naiad in the conjunctival sac of *Nyctimistes daymani.* The picture shows a section through the conjunctival sac (the space under the eyelids) of a New Guinea frog, and might suggest a parasite invading the frog by way of the eye. The worm in question, however, is not a parasitic type but a harmless freshwater worm which could only have entered the frog's eye accidentally. It is remarkable to notice that, in spite of the fact that the worm has bristles, no defence reaction on the part of the frog can be seen. The defences of lower animals against agents of all kinds which threaten their health are often found extremely insufficient and ineffective. Photo: Elkan.

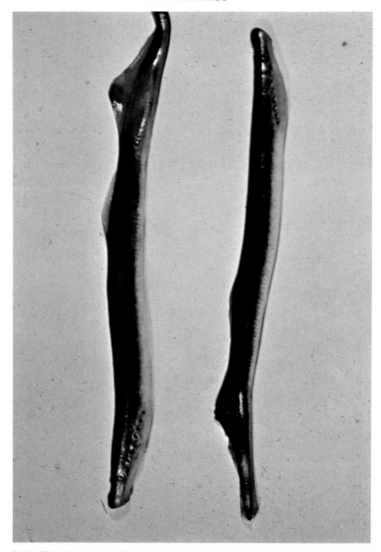

296. The lamprey *(Lampetra fluviatilis)* attaches itself to the skin of weakened or captive fish and lives on their substance. Heavy losses through infestation with lampreys occurred in the Great Lakes of North America.

IV. GENETIC DISORDERS
AND
TRAUMA

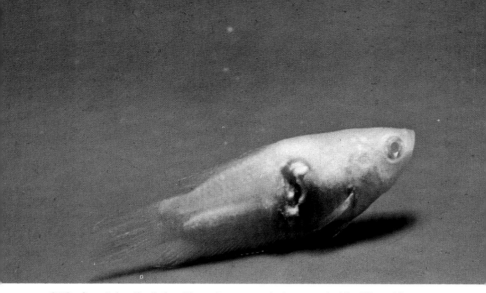

297. An albinotic fish with red eyes and ulcerated skin. The skin condition may be due to bacterial infection, vitamin deficiency or water pollution. Photo: Frickhinger.

298. Congenital anomalies in salmon parr.

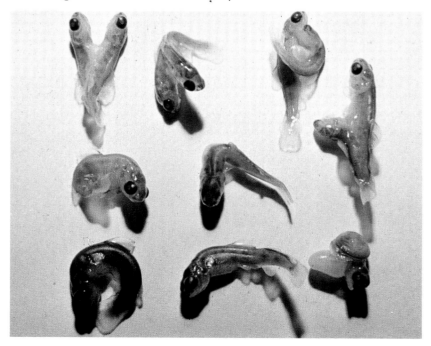

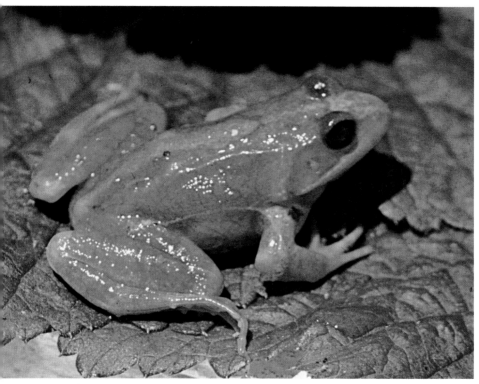

299. Amelanotic grass frog *(Rana temporaria)*. The more profusely an animal species breeds, the more likely it is that malformations will occur. Deficiencies in pigmentation in amphibians and reptiles are not very common, but have been described from many localities. The specimen shown cannot be described as an albino because the black pigmented layer (tapetum) which makes the eye into a camera obscura is well developed. The lack of pigmentation has a negative survival value because the orange-colored frog is much more easily spotted than its well camouflaged brothers. Photo: Elkan.

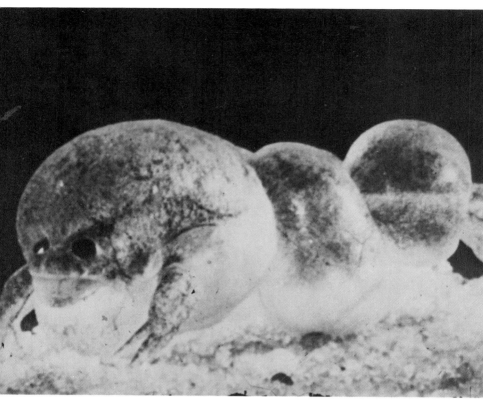

300. Hydropic young *Xenopus laevis.* Normally the lymph sacs which in amphibians lie between the skin and the body are emptied by two sets of lymph hearts, one situated in the coccygeal, the other in the thoracic region. As a consequence of maldevelopment these lymph hearts may be deficient. As a result the serous lining of the lymph sacs continues to produce lymph, but the sacs cannot empty themselves. Thus the condition of lymphatic hydrops develops. Eventually the skin of the frog becomes so thin that the muscles can be seen plainly through it. The condition is fatal. Photo: Elkan.

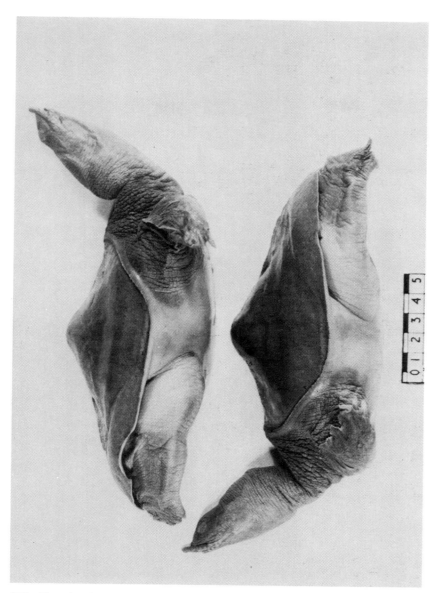

301. Vertebral deformity (kyphosis) in a Nile soft-shelled turtle
(Trionyx triunguis). Deformed animals may, under favorable conditions, reach maturity. The turtle with the deformed spinal column
shown here did not die in consequence of this deformity, but by
electrocution when it became involved with an electric heater.
Photo: Elkan.

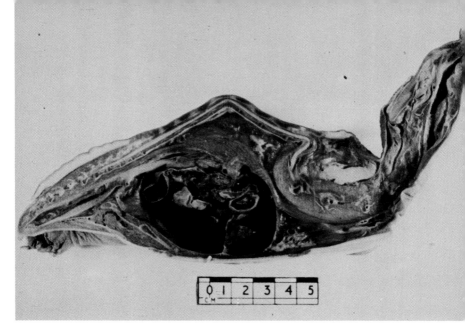

302. To show the relations of the main organs, the specimen was frozen and then cut along the mid-line with a band saw. It can be seen that the kyphosis created an empty space which was not taken up by any of the other organic systems. The empty space contained only fluid and some connective tissue fibers. Photo: Elkan.

303. Nile soft-shell *Trionyx triunguis* with kyphotic spine. A sagittal midline section in which: A = penis, B = brain, C = cloaca, F = fat deposit, G = bronchus, H = region of heart, I = intestine, K = kyphotic vertebrae, L = liver, O = oral cavity, P = pelvic bone, R = retractor muscle of neck, S = space created by the kyphosis, T = tongue, U = region of urinary bladder. Photo: Elkan.

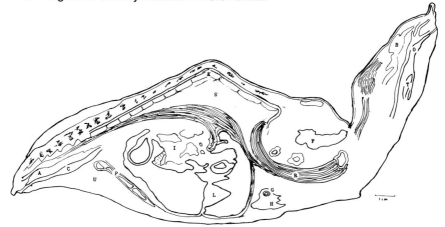

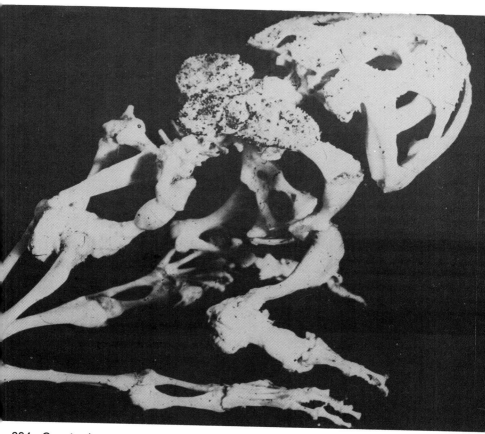

304. *Ceratophrys ornatus* with multiple fractures. Accidents happen even in the life of frogs. When the skeleton of this large Brazilian specimen was examined, it was found that the right ilium (part of the pelvis) and the right radio-ulna (forearm) showed bones crushed by severe trauma and left to heal as best they could without the benefit of a surgeon. Since the accident must have occurred in the Brazilian jungle, it was probably due to an encounter with a predator. It is difficult to understand how the frog survived an assault of this severity and how it could continue life with a complete ankylosis (bony fusion) of both the hip and the elbow joints on the right. Note, incidentally, the large bony dorsal shield typical of this genus but not found in ordinary frogs. Photo: Elkan.

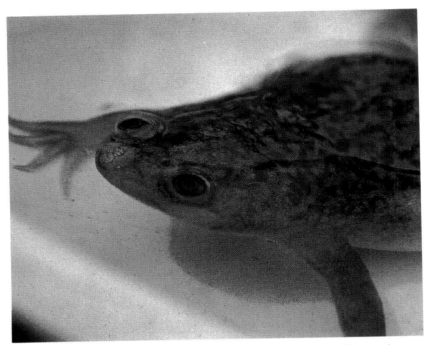

305. *Xenopus laevis* with injured nasal region. Newly caught specimens sometimes make frequent and violent attempts to escape and, in the process, injure the rostral (nasal) region of the head. In spite of the pain that this must cause, these attempts may be repeated until an ulcer develops at the injured spot. Since the healing power of the frog's skin is poor, such an ulcer may lead to sepsis (general infection) and the death of 'the specimen. Newly captured specimens should be kept in the dark and in containers giving them the least possible chance to injure themselves. Photo: Elkan.

V. NUTRITIONAL DISORDERS

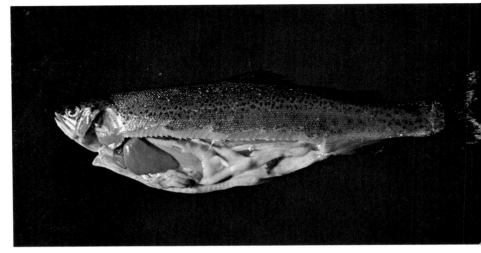

306. Lipoid degeneration of the liver of a rainbow trout *(Salmo gairdneri).* Note the pale discoloration of the liver.

307. Liver of a fish suffering from fatty degeneration and biliary infiltration.

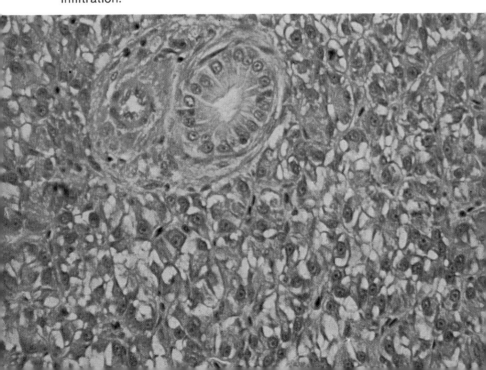

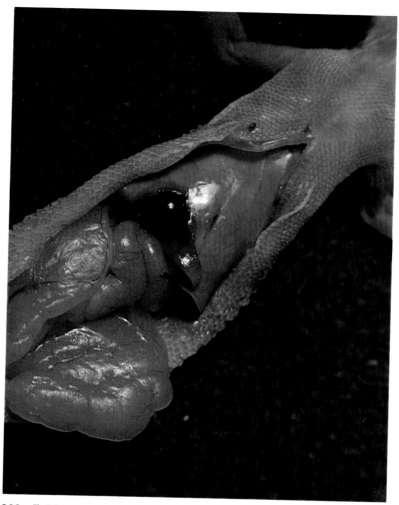

308. *Eublepharis fasciolatus* is a gecko found in southern Asia. The condition shown is never seen in freshly caught animals, but is commonly found at the necropsy of specimens which have died in captivity. If an animal is given more food than it needs, if it no longer has to search for food and has neither incentive nor opportunity for exercise, fat accumulates in the body, and the liver eventually presents the picture seen in those of artificially fed geese. It is never easy to gauge exactly how much food small captive animals need. One does not like to err on the low side, but it equally harms the animal to feed it more than it would get in a good day's (or night's) hunting in its natural habitat. Photo: Elkan.

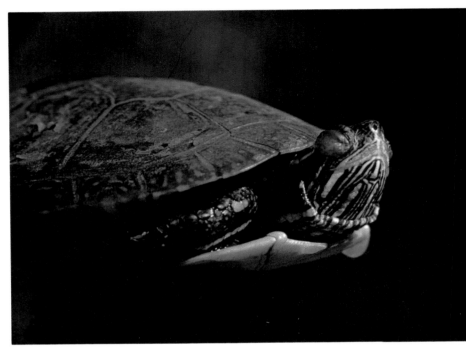

309. Typical cases of vitamin deficiency are seen only in captive animals which have, over a lengthy period, received an unsuitable diet. For short periods they store a sufficient amount of vitamins in their liver. In lower vertebrates avitaminosis occurs most commonly in the small turtles which are slowly starved to an early death on the diet of ant eggs usually recommended by the dealers. Their normal diet consists of live pond snails, insects and plants. To replace these a carefully balanced diet of proteins and calcium is required. The disease shows itself first in a swelling of the eyelids. As soon as the lids swell so much that the animal can no longer open the eyes, it stops feeding and the prognosis from that moment onward is hopeless. Treatment is made more difficult by the fact that vitamin A, which is most urgently required, is not soluble in water and would have to be given by force feeding the small turtle, which is extremely difficult. Photo: Elkan.

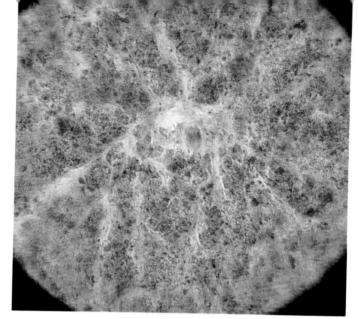

310. This lizard *(Iguana iguana),* which had been kept in captivity for several years, was found to have an enlarged, pale grey liver. The color of a normal liver is brownish-red. The picture shows the fat droplets (stained orange) which fill the liver cells and which are far in excess of what the animal needs. Photo: Elkan.

311. Avitaminosis in *Pseudemys scripta elegans.* Photo: Elkan.

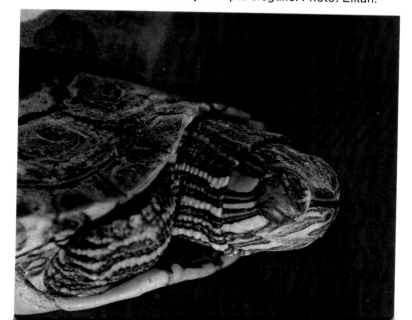

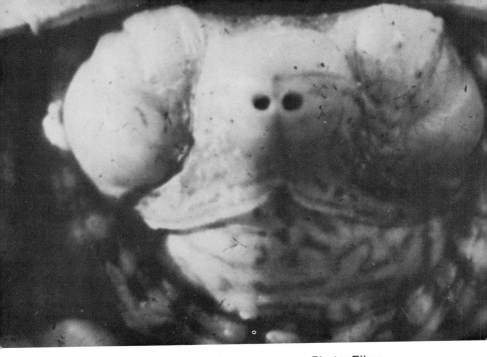

312 — 313. Avitaminosis in *Clemmys leprosa*. Photo: Elkan.

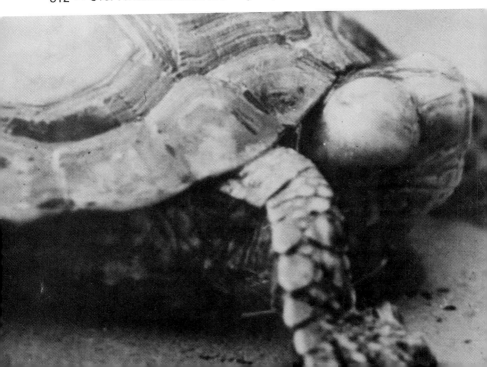

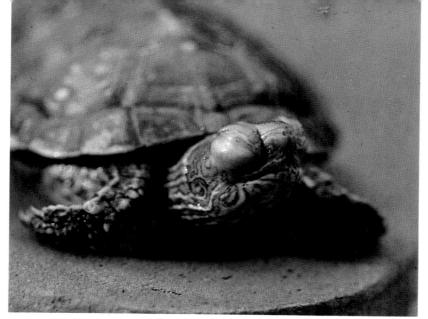

314. Avitaminosis in *Clemmys leprosa*. Photo: Elkan.

315. Dissection of the head of a *Chrysemys picta* with avitaminosis. The swelling of the eyelids is caused by a degeneration of the Harderian gland, the ducts of which become blocked. As the picture shows, the swollen eyelids eventually meet and cover the eye so that the turtle becomes blind. The eyeball itself, however, is unaffected. Photo: Elkan.

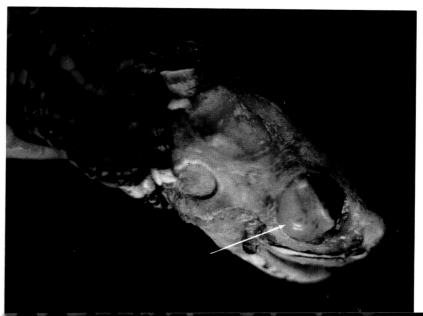

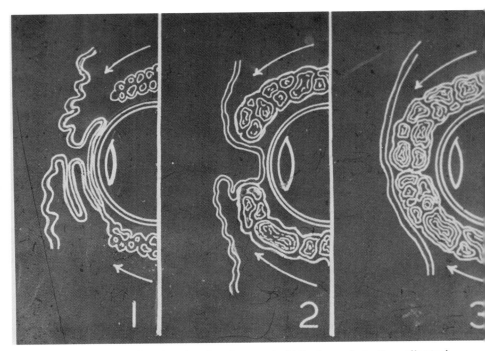

316. Diagram showing the development of blindness in turtles affected
by avitaminosis A. Figure 1 shows the conjunctival sac and the
nictitating membrane in their normal state. The lacrimal glands are
well set back. In Figure 2 the lacrimal glands have started to enlarge
and to fill in the nictitating membrane. The eyelids can only be
partially opened. In Figure 3 the lacrimal glands have enlarged so
much that the whole of the conjunctival space is filled in. The eye can
no longer be opened and the turtle is blind. Note that during the whole
of this development the eyeball is not affected and remains completely
normal. Photo: Elkan.

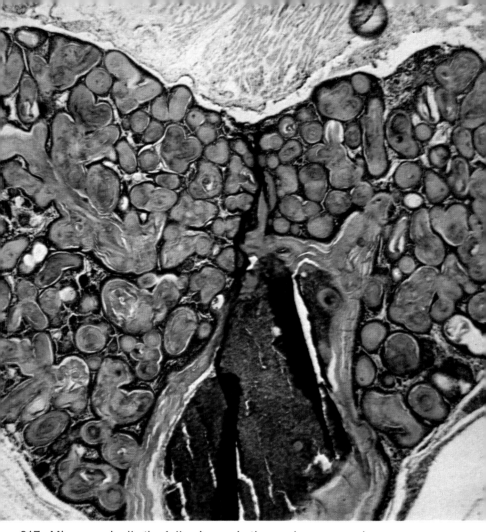

317. Microscopically the following main tissue changes can be
observed in avitaminosis of turtles. a) Metaplasia of the epithelium in
the Harderian gland, the kidneys and the ureters. The normal columnar
epithelium changes into stratified epithelium. b) Hyperkeratinization.
The abnormal epithelium produces masses of keratin which block the
ducts and prevent even the parts of the organ which may be normal
from functioning. c) An intensive eosinophilia. There appear in the
bloodstream large numbers of leucocytes which stain heavily with
eosin. These eosinophils conglomerate particularly in the lymphatic
spaces around excretory ducts (liver, pancreas, etc.) and in the
interstitial tissue of the kidney. The picture shows *Chrysemys picta*
with metaplasia and hyperkeratinization of the Harderian gland.
Photo: Elkan.

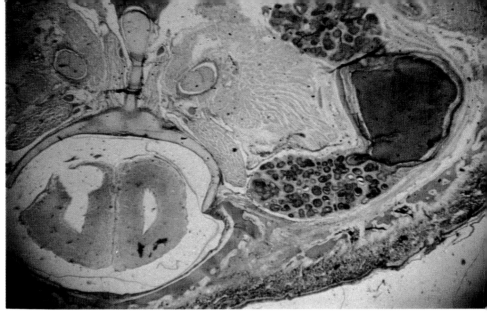

318. Avitaminosis in *Chinemys reevesii.* Note the large accumulation of keratin between two lobes of the degenerating Harderian gland. Photo: Elkan.

319. *Pseudemys scripta* with avitaminosis A. Note the accumulation of eosinophils in the interstitial tissue of the kidney. Photo: Elkan.

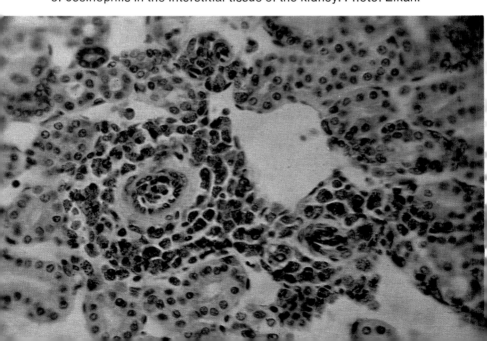

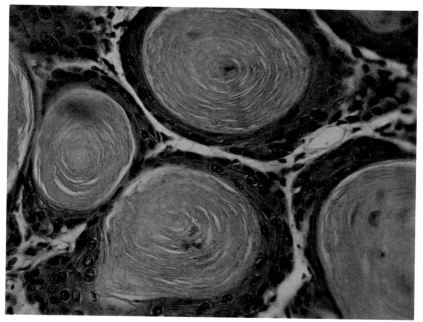

320. *Chinemys reevesii* with avitaminosis showing metaplasia and hyperkeratinization of the Harderian gland. Photo: Elkan.

321. Avitaminotic *Pseudemys scripta* showing accumulations of eosinophils in the kidney. Photo: Elkan.

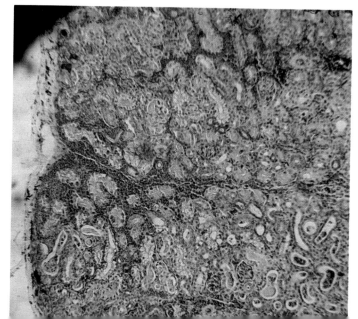

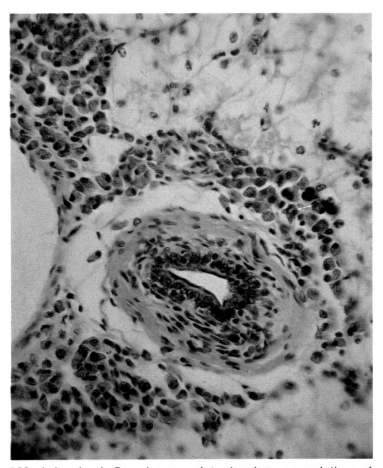

322. Avitaminotic *Pseudemys scripta* showing accumulations of eosinophils in lymphatic sheaths of the hepatic excretory ducts. Photo: Elkan.

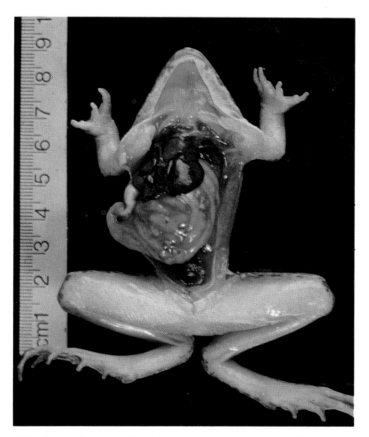

323. *Rana tigrina* with distension of the stomach. It is not advisable to overfeed small animals before sending them on long journeys. This small Indian frog was placed in a cotton bag together with several others. Before the start of the long journey to England it was allowed to eat as much as it liked. It was, however, unable to digest all of this food so it fermented in the stomach. The stomach became distended and in turn prevented the frog from breathing. Lack of space probably was a contributory factor, and all of the animals died. At necropsy the frog's stomach contained thirty-seven mealworms. Photo: Elkan.

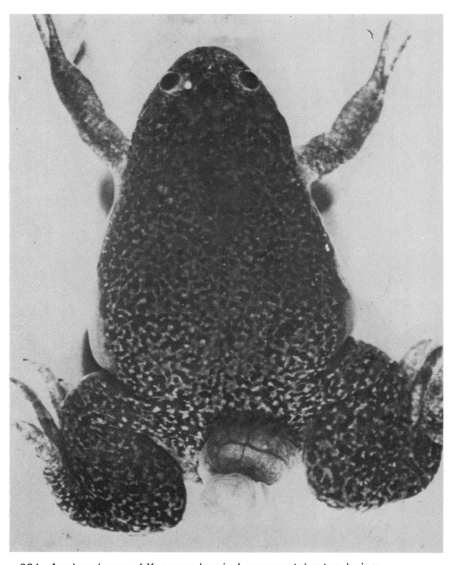

324. Anal prolapse of *Xenopus laevis.* Lower vertebrates, being unable to chew their food, have to swallow it whole. If they are hungry they may well attempt to swallow relatively large prey. This happens particularly in frogs which have a disproportionately wide mouth. The egestion of the indigestible part of such meals may present difficulties and cause the prolapse of part of the large intestine. Treatment of the condition is unrewarding. In most cases, if the animal is starved for a period, the prolapse subsides spontaneously. Only rarely does it lead to such complications as local ulceration or intestinal obstruction. Photo: Elkan.

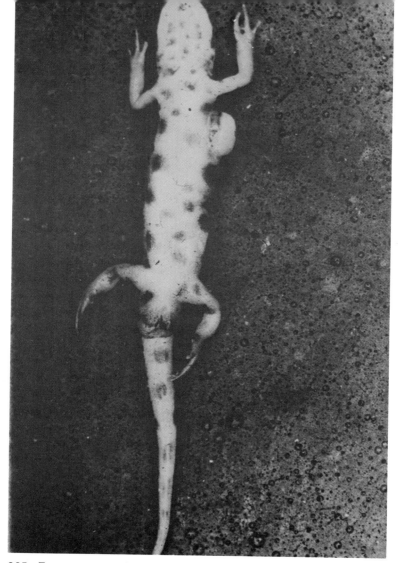

325. For reasons which we do not understand, even wild animals on occasion eat something entirely unsuitable. The newt *(Triturus vulgaris)* shown here was moribund when caught. It could be seen that there was a large gap in the lateral body wall on one side. The cause for this injury became clear when microscopic sections were made through the whole specimen. It could then be seen that the newt's stomach was full of decaying vegetable matter. This fermentation had produced gas which had distended the stomach to such an extent that it had ruptured the body wall, thus producing a gastric hernia. If this newt had not been caught it would undoubtedly have died very shortly. Normally newts are carnivorous. Photo: Elkan.

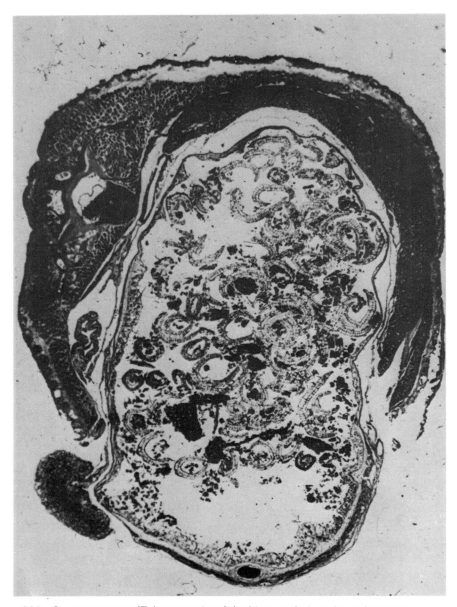

326. Common newt *(Triturus vulgaris)* with gastric hernia and rupture of the body wall. The stomach, distended by fermenting vegetable matter, has burst through the lateral body wall, a condition which, in a higher animal, would be fatal. The newt survived. Photo: Elkan.

VI. ENVIRONMENTAL DISEASES
AND
HEMATOLOGICAL DISEASES

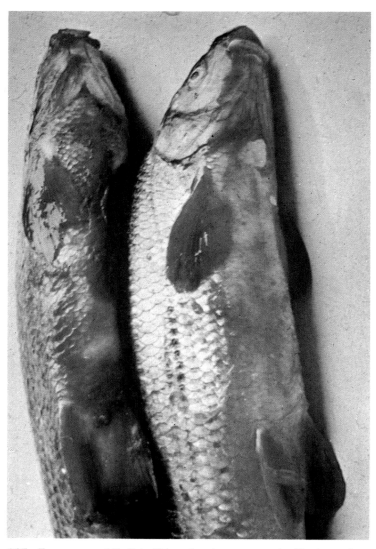

327. European whitefish *(Chondrostoma nasus)* with dermal ulceration due to water pollution.

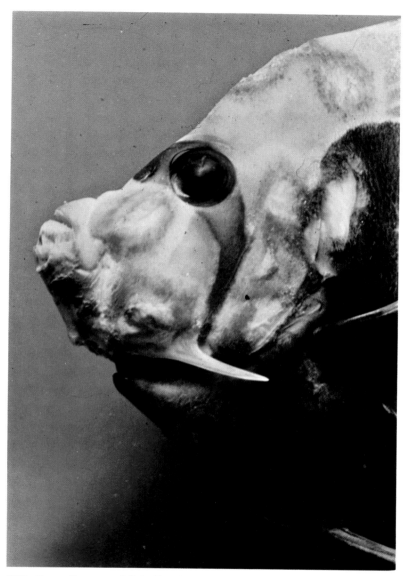

328. Sore disease of fish. Patches of inflammation widely distributed. Conditions of this kind are frequently caused by pollutants which damage the skin, certain bacteria (aeromonads) and nutritional deficiencies. Photo: Frickhinger.

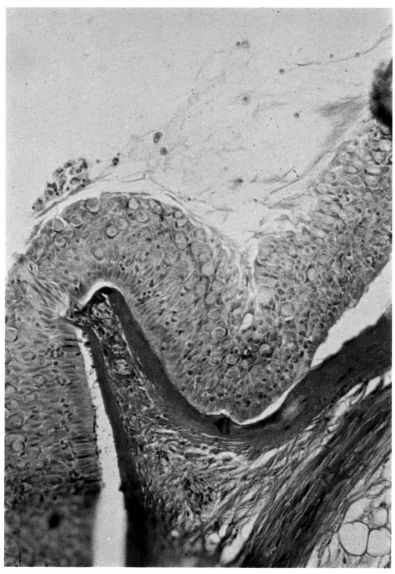

329. Section through the skin of a healthy fish.

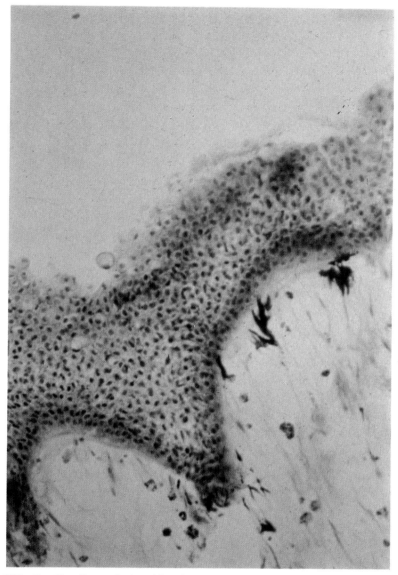

330. Section through the skin of a fish damaged by oil pollution.

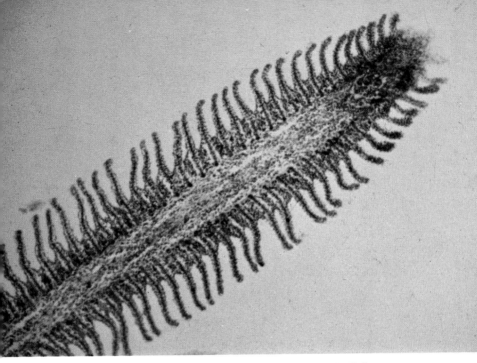

331. Section through the gills of an undamaged whitefish (*Chrondrostoma*).

332. Damaged gills of a fish. Note the oedematous tips with mucus producing cells.

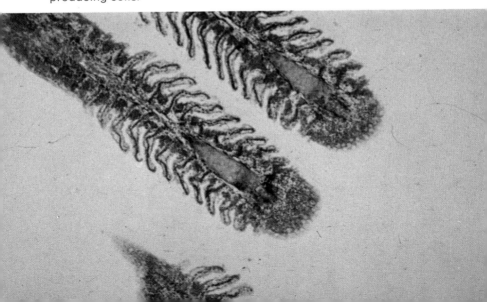

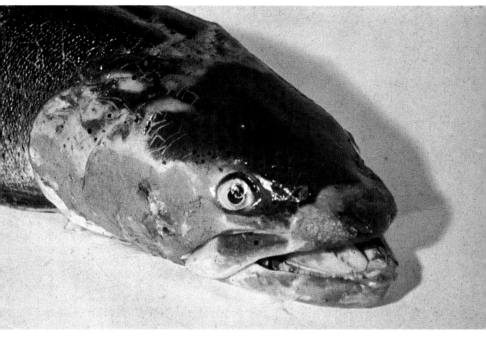

333. Huchen *(Hucho hucho),* the Danubian salmon, with ulcerative dermal necrosis complicated by fungal infection of the head.

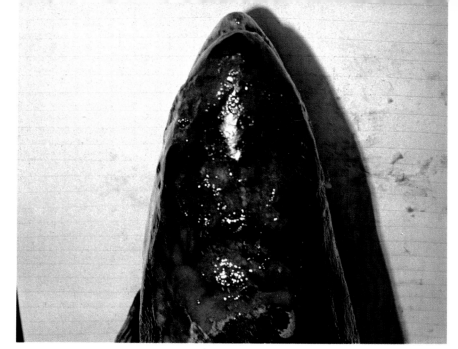

334. Ulcerative dermal necrosis (UDN) on the head of an Atlantic salmon *(Salmo salar).*

335. Grayling *(Thymallus thymallus)* with signs of ulcerative dermal necrosis.

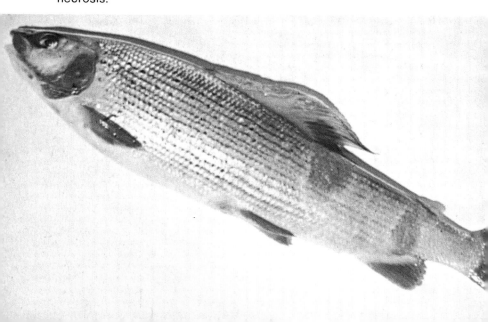

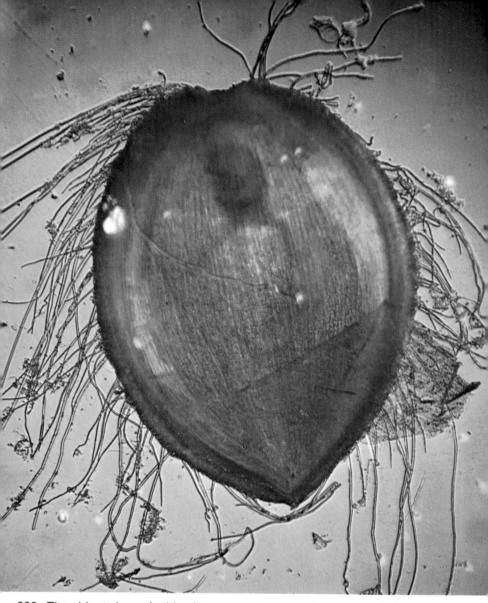

336. The object shown in this picture was discovered, accompanied by two others of the same kind, in the pharynx of a frog. In spite of its suggestive appearance, this foreign body is not a parasite and it is not even of a zoological but of a botanical nature. So far it has been possible to identify this tentatively as a hair-covered seed of a plant of the genus *Ruellia* (Acanthaceae). The textbooks report that the seeds anchor themselves with the aid of the hairs, which swell when they get wet. The frog seems to have been unable to dislodge these presumably irritating bodies from its throat. Photo: Elkan.

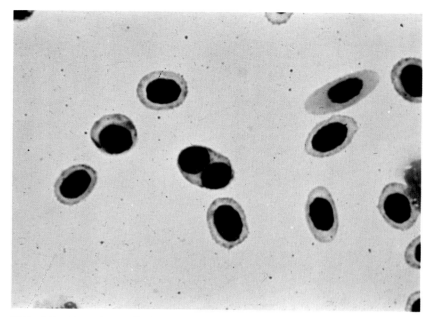

337. Atlantic salmon *(Salmo salar)* with microcytic anemia.

338. Packed red cell volume (hematocrit) from normal fish at top and from an anemic fish on the bottom.

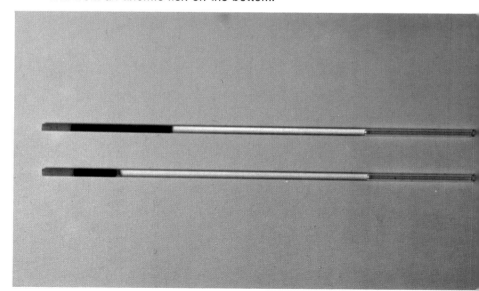

VII. NEOPLASTIC DISEASES

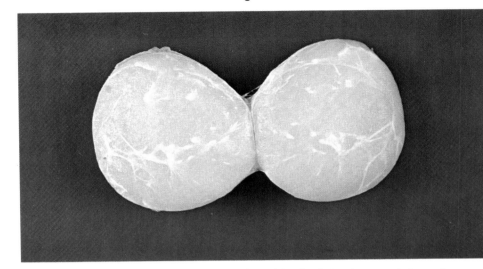

339. A well circumscribed lipoma found in the lateral musculature of a largemouth bass. Note the white connective tissue stroma throughout the tumor. Photo: Mawdesley-Thomas.

340. One of the vesicle lobes of the urinary bladder is transformed into a solid tumor. Histologically it was found to be a fibroma (connective tissue tumor) and it is doubtful that it killed the host *(Bufo bufo)*. Photo: Elkan.

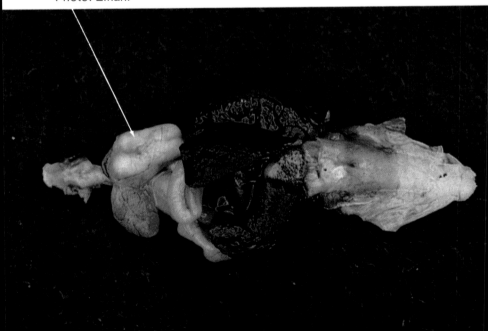

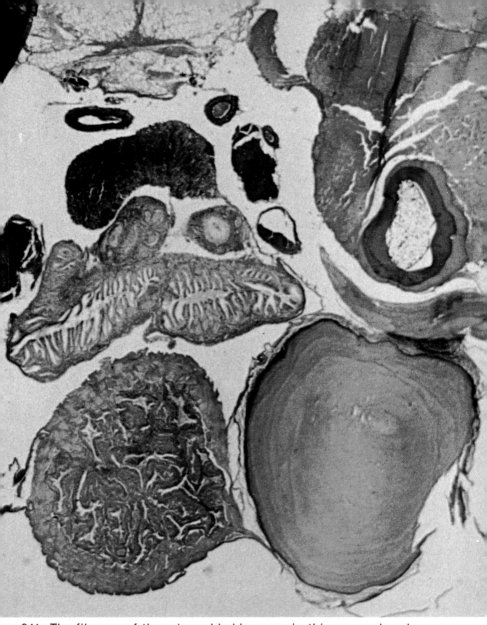

341. The fibroma of the urinary bladder was, in this case, placed so that it obstructed the outflow of urine. The bladder, in consequence, became more and more hypertrophic (overgrowth of muscle tissue). The solid tumor occupies the right part of the picture, and the hypertrophic bladder the left. The other structures seen are parts of the frog's intestine. (Van Gieson stain). Photo: Elkan.

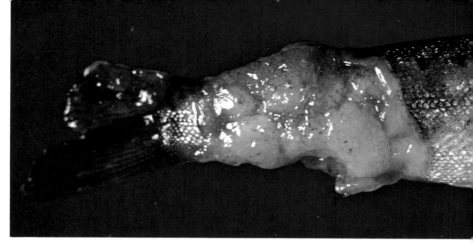

342. Papilloma on the caudal peduncle of an Atlantic salmon
(Salmo salar).

343. Carp *(Cyprinus carpio)* are extensively bred for food in European
fish ponds. It is essential that the fish coming to market should have
no blemishes whatsoever. Unfortunately their skin is occasionally
affected by small warty growths which, on close inspection, reveal
themselves as dermal papillomata. It may be more than a coincidence
that the same fresh fish are frequently found infested with fish lice
(Argulus sp.), and it seems very likely that, just as with ticks in reptiles,
the fish lice transmit viruses which, when introduced into the skin by
the bite of the louse, elicit the growth of the tumors. In the case shown
here the papilloma arose on the operculum (gill cover) of the fish.
Photo: Elkan.

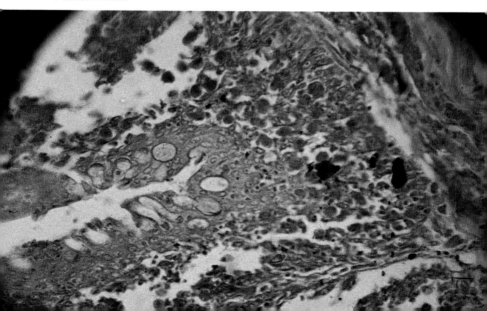

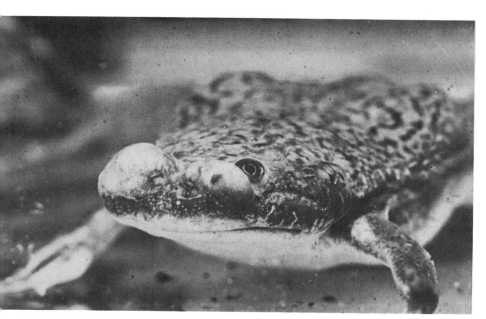

344. Facial tumors are particularly common in animals which try repeatedly to escape through a glass pane which they do not see. There must, however, be additional causes for these lesions around the nose since they were also observed in *Xenopus* sp. kept in steel tanks. The picture shows a typical case where benign fibromata developed around both nostrils. They did not seriously affect the toad. Photo: Elkan.

345. Papilloma of the nostril of *Xenopus laevis*. This tumor, which at first sight looks harmless, is in fact premalignant. Photo: Elkan.

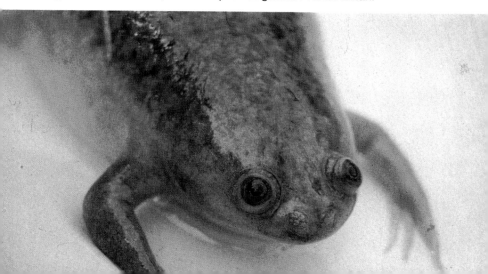

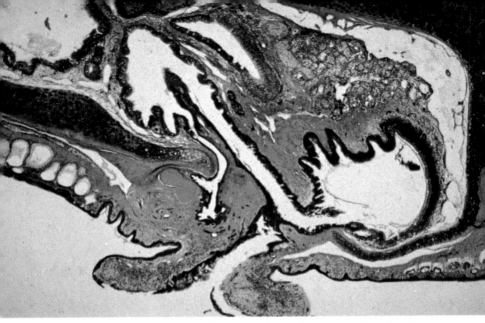

346. The nasal papilloma of *Xenopus laevis* has a peculiar structure resembling in some parts a glandular carcinoma. It has invaded the subcutaneous tissue but has not produced any metastases. Although little of the tumor showed on the surface, the afflicted toad refused to feed and had to be killed. Photo: Elkan.

347. The nasal papilloma of the *Xenopus laevis* is seen to be a melanopapilloma. Photo: Elkan.

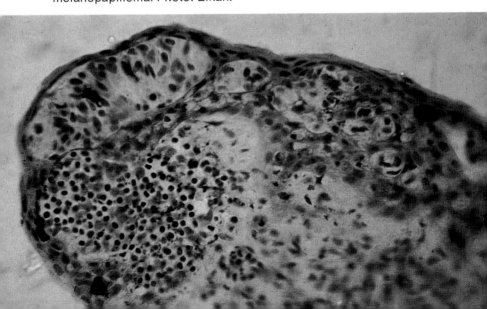

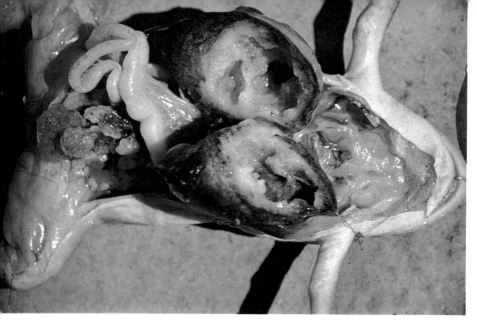

348. This comparatively large but benign glandular tumor (adenoma) gradually destroyed the liver of the host *(Xenopus laevis)*. Photo: Elkan.

349. This adenoma from the liver of *Xenopus laevis* eventually outgrew its blood supply and became necrotic centrally. There was no sign of cancerous degeneration and no metastases were found. The frog probably died from hepatic insufficiency. Photo: Elkan.

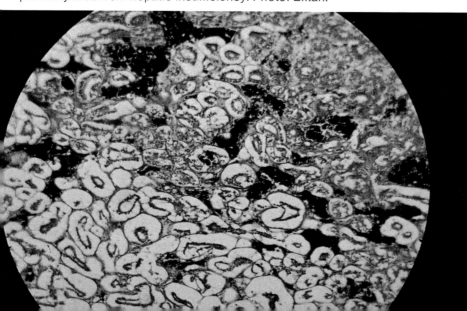

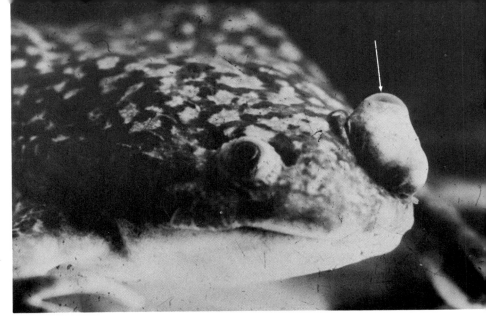

350. The ophthalmic adenoma does not arise from the nostril but from the eye. It arises, in fact, deep in the eye socket, pushing the eyeball a considerable distance away from its normal condition. The tumor shown must have stretched the optic nerve, but although the toad must have been blind on the affected side, it continued to feed. Eventually the tumor protruded outwards and inwards obstructing part of the mouth of the host *(Xenopus laevis)* as well. Photo: Elkan.

351. Ophthalmic adenoma in *Xenopus laevis.* Photo: Elkan.

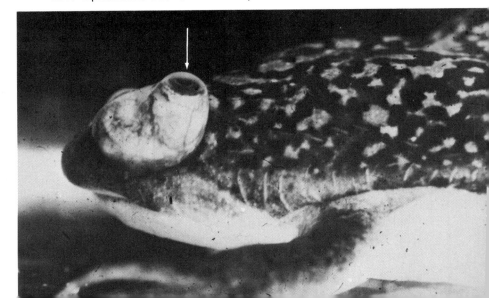

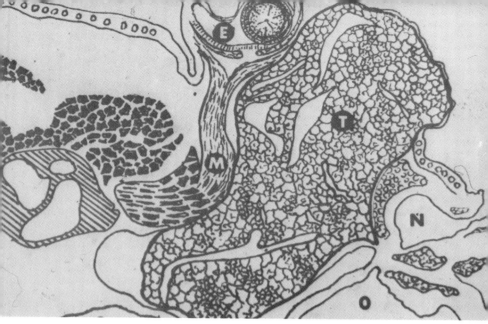

352. Diagram of section through an ophthalmic adenoma in *Xenopus laevis*. Sections proved the tumor to be an adenoma arising from the Harderian gland. The pressure exerted by the growing tumor displaced the eyeball. No metastases could be found. E, eye; M, ocular retractor muscle; N, nostril; O, oral cavity; T, tumor. Photo: Elkan.

353. Embryonic tumors in lower vertebrates arise more frequently from the kidney than from other organs. Why this should be so we do not know. The picture shows a nephroblastoma which occurred in a rainbow trout (*Salmo gairdneri*). Photo: Harshbarger.

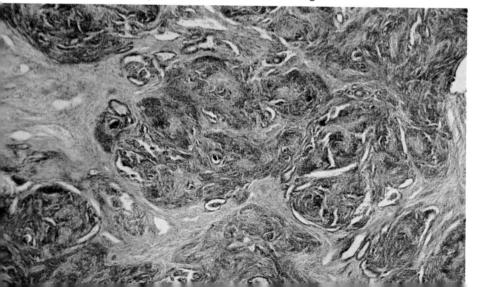

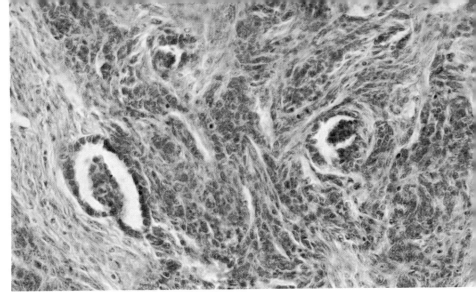

354. Nephroblastomas grow to a considerable size, and even if they do not metastasize they interfere severely with the host's normal metabolism by displacing the surrounding intestines. Photo: Harshbarger.

355. Just as in human pathology, tumors due to embryonic maldevelopment occur in lower animals. They may lie dormant and become obvious only relatively late in the life of the individual. The kidney is one of the organs more commonly affected, and although the tumor is not malignant it may, by its growth, interfere so much with the functioning of the intestines that it becomes a danger to life. Photo: Elkan.

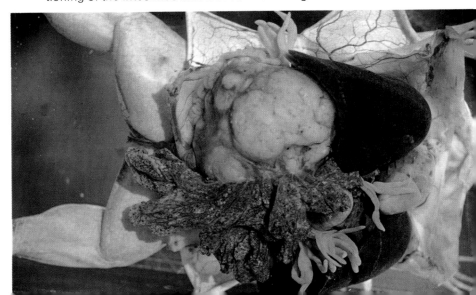

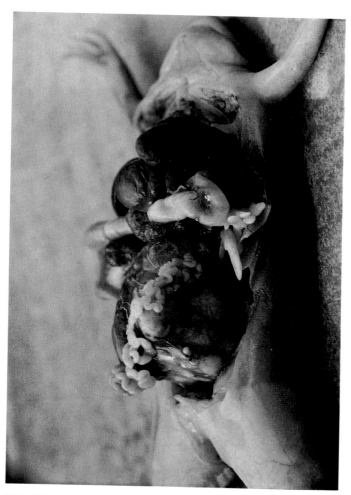

356. The nephroblastoma, when fully grown, seems to fill the body cavity of the host *(Xenopus laevis)*. In fact, it arises retroperitoneally since the kidneys lie outside the main body cavity, and in growing the tumor pushes and displaces all the other viscera forward against the ventral body wall. The lateral view shows the visceral displacement. The left oviduct, which normally lies deep in the pelvis, is seen lying on top of the tumor. Photo: Elkan.

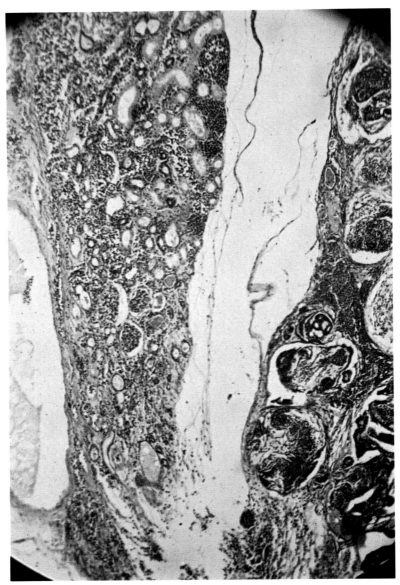

357. The kidney in which a nephroblastoma arises (left half of picture) becomes so compressed by the expanding tumor that it ceases to function. The right half of the picture shows part of the tumor which contains no recognizable structures. Photo: Elkan.

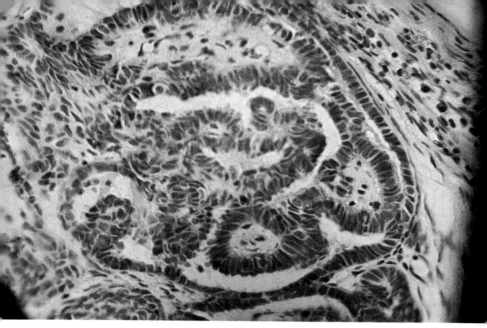

358. Microscopically the nephroblastoma in *Xenopus laevis* makes frustrated attempts at the formation of normal renal elements like tubules and glomeruli. In some instances the disorganized tissue almost seems to succeed in producing at least normal epithelium, but no part of the tumor ever produces functional renal tissue. Photo: Elkan.

359. An unidentified tumor on the head of an anabantid fish.

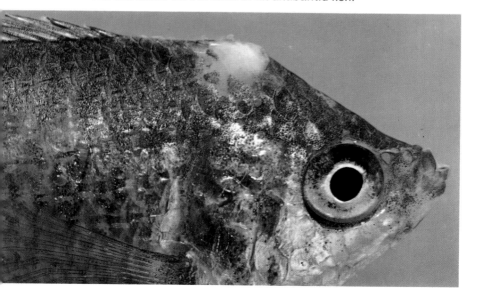

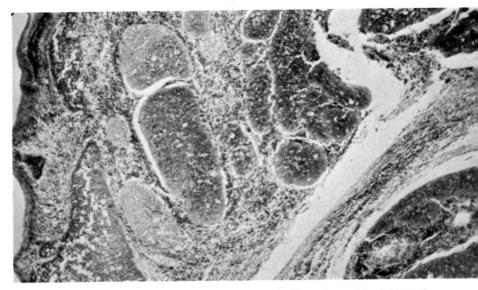

360. Basal cell carcinoma in a golden orfe *(Leuciscus idus)*. Note the "island" appearance of the infiltrating cells. Photo: Mawdesley-Thomas.

361. Squamous cell carcinoma on the head of a gudgeon. Note the local cell nests surrounded by marked fibroblastic response. Photo: Mawdesley-Thomas.

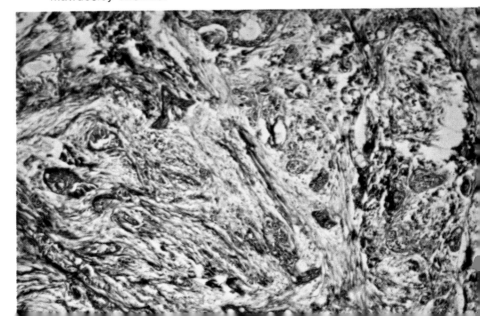

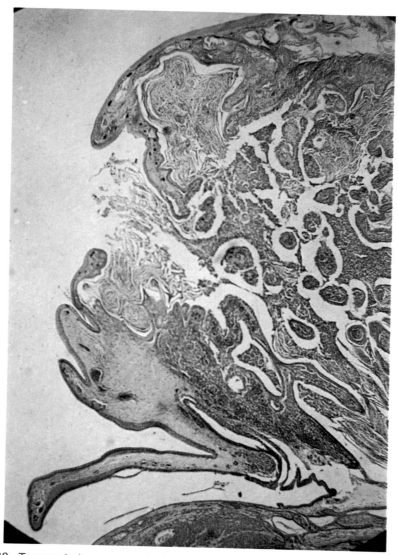

362. Tumors in lower animals, in common with those occurring in man and the higher vertebrates, occur more frequently in old than in young specimens. Analagous to what we see in elderly human patients, frogs too may get a slow growing cancerous ulcer of the face. The picture shows the break in the normal skin, the ulcer derived from the local destruction and part of the cancerous growth which has already invaded deeper parts of the head. A tumor of this kind, even if it is slow growing, must be regarded as a malignant epithelioma because it may destroy any organ in its way and set up metastases anywhere. The tumor in the picture occurred in *Rana temporaria.* Photo: Elkan.

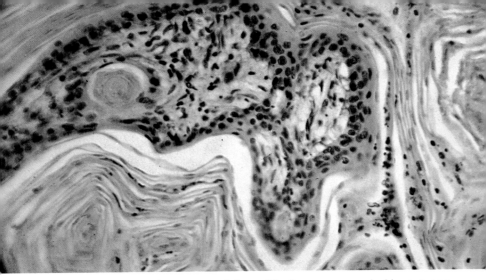

363. The picture shows part of the epithelioma surrounded by masses of keratin destroying and displacing tissues in the deeper layers of the frog's *(Rana temporaria)* head. The dark colored strands of atypical epithelial cells are unable to form any normal type of tissue but destroy any normal cells in their way. Photo: Elkan.

364. Epithelioma taken from the face of *Rana temporaria*. Photo: Elkan.

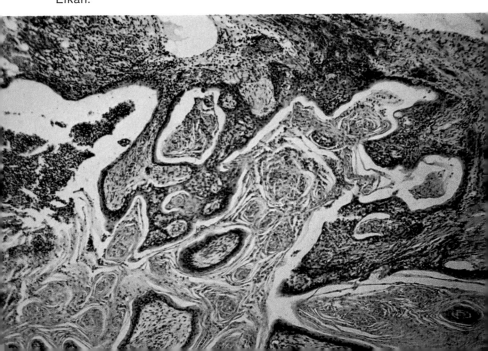

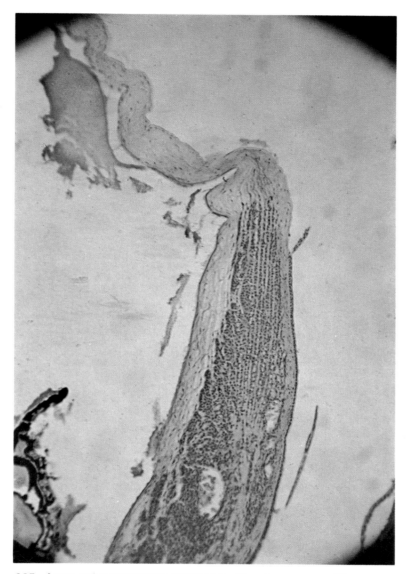

365. Among the structures invaded by the cancerous epithelioma was the eye of *Rana temporaria*. The cornea, consisting
of fairly tough layers of fibers, presented an obstacle to the
advancing tumor cells. The picture shows the tumor advancing
between the layers of the cornea. Photo: Elkan.

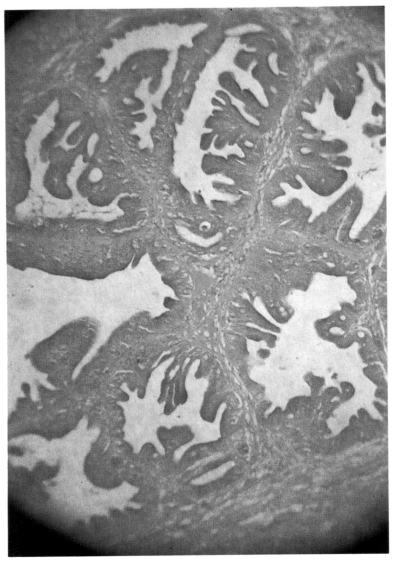

366. Glandular tumors may occur in many organs. Some are relatively harmless, but an adenocarcinoma occurring in the renal pelvis may obstruct the flow of urine. It may also, if it grows to a large size, injure neighboring organs by displacing them. The tumor shown here is a papillary adenocarcinoma taken from *Boa constrictor,* a species which seems to be more prone to this disease than other snakes. Photo: Elkan.

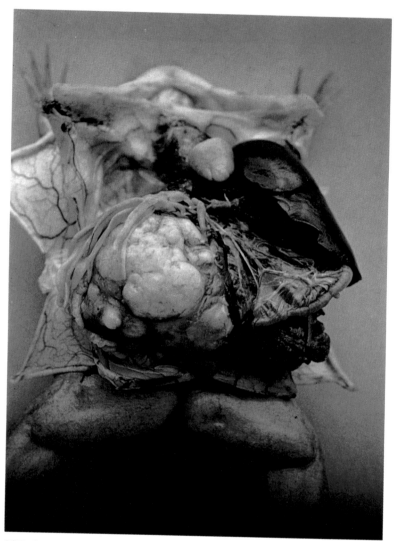

367. Malignant tumors in lower vertebrates, particularly in amphibians and reptiles, are rare. The kidney takes first place among the organs which may be affected by malignant growths. The picture shows a case of renal carcinoma in *Xenopus laevis* which has reached a considerable size and has produced many metastases and invasive growths. It never fails to amaze the observer how long lower animals can survive even when afflicted by a cancerous condition which must seriously interfere with the function of some of the vital organs. Photo: Elkan.

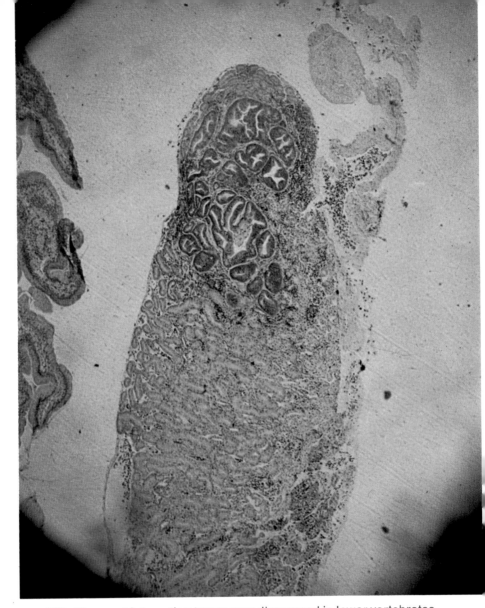

368. The most interesting tumor ever discovered in lower vertebrates is undoubtedly the renal adenocarcinoma first described by Lucke in 1934 in *Rana pipiens*. A whole library of papers has since been written on this tumor, which proved most suitable for laboratory investigations into the nature of cancer. About 2.7% of frogs caught in their natural habitat show the tumor, which grows rapidly, even under laboratory conditions. Photo: Elkan.

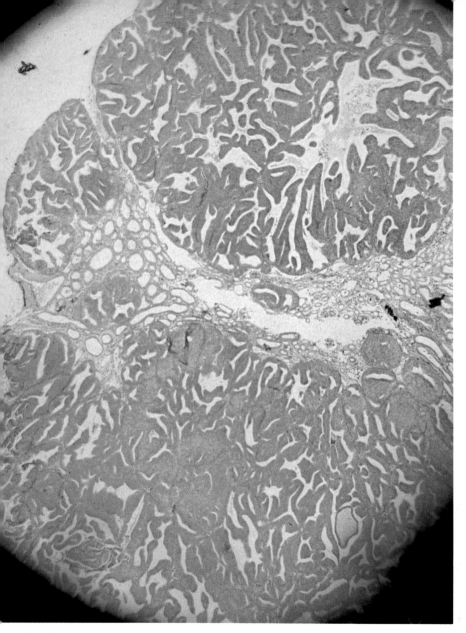

369. The adenocarcinoma in *Rana pipiens* may assume the shape of an adenoma or it may appear as an unorganized (anaplastic) mass. It always shows many mitotic figures indicating rapid cell division and soon produces secondary deposits. The subject has been reviewed by Rafferty (1964, Cancer Research 24: 169-185). Photo: Rafferty.

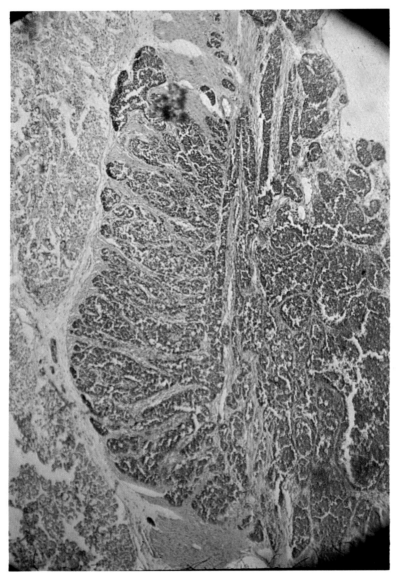

370. Spontaneous anaplastic carcinoma of the stomach in *Xenopus laevis*. Tumors of this kind must be considered as extraordinarily rare. Although thousands of frogs are annually used for classwork dissection, no other case has come to light. Photo: Elkan.

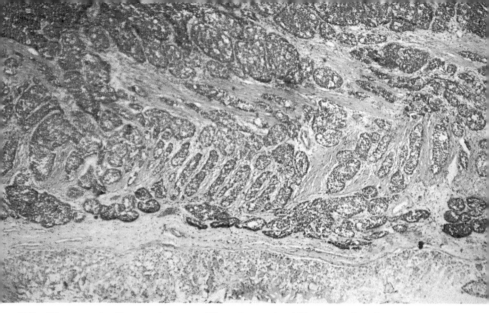

371. The anaplastic carcinoma of the stomach of *Xenopus laevis* probably arose in the gastric glands. It does not imitate the glandular structure, but is completely structureless. Photo: Elkan.

372. Anaplastic carcinoma of the stomach which has invaded and largely destroyed the pancreas of *Xenopus laevis*. Photo: Elkan.

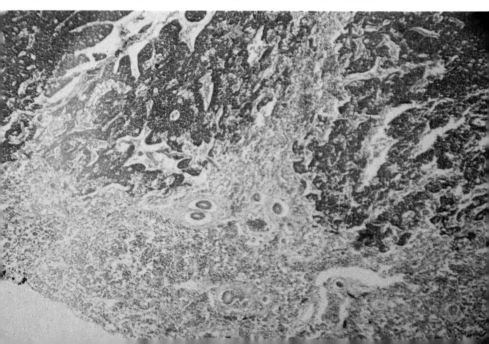

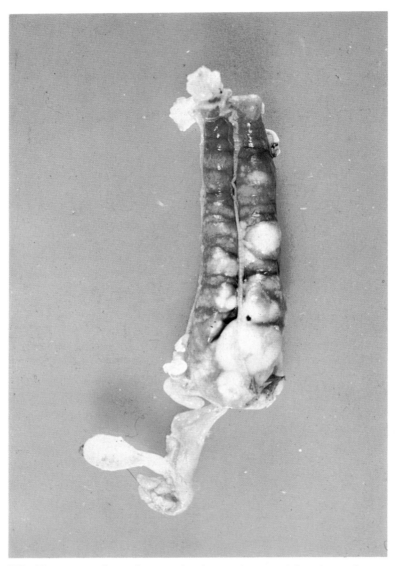

373. Metastases from the anaplastic carcinoma of the stomach were found in the kidney and in the wall of the urinary bladder of *Xenopus laevis*. Both organs were reduced in size and could no longer function. Note that it could not be decided by naked eye inspection whether a kidney, found in this condition, was affected by cancer, tuberculosis or a fungal infection. Photo: Elkan.

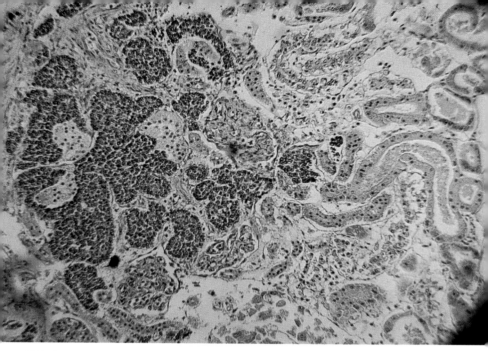

374. Metastases from the anaplastic carcinoma of the stomach in the kidney of *Xenopus laevis*. Photo: Elkan.

375. Melanosarcoma in a cod. Note that the surrounding skeletal muscle is infiltrated. Photo: Mawdesley-Thomas.

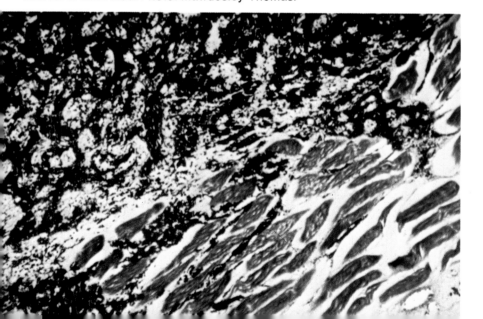

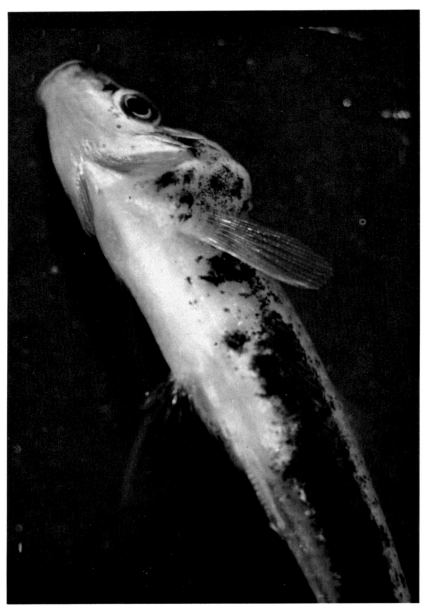

376. Melanosarcoma in a platy *(Xiphophorus maculatus)*. This is a malignant rapidly growing dark colored tumor of migrating giant melanophores.

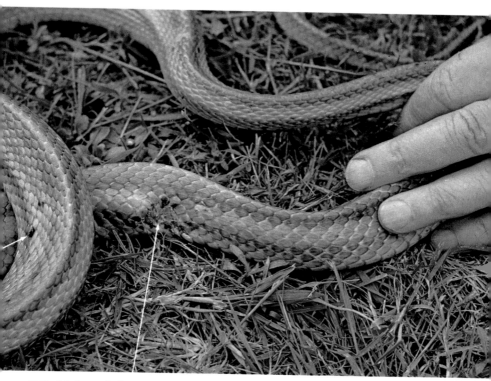

377. Melanosis is a cancerous condition arising from the pigment-bearing cells (melanocytes) in the skin, the eye or elsewhere. Because of its rapid growth, its insidious spreading and its power of destruction, it is considered as one of the most malignant tumors known. Photo: Grimstone.

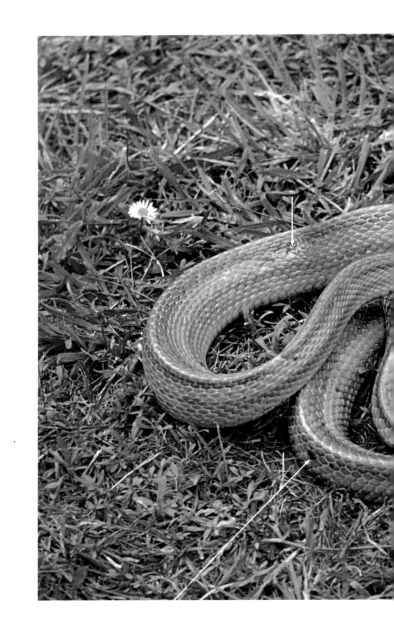

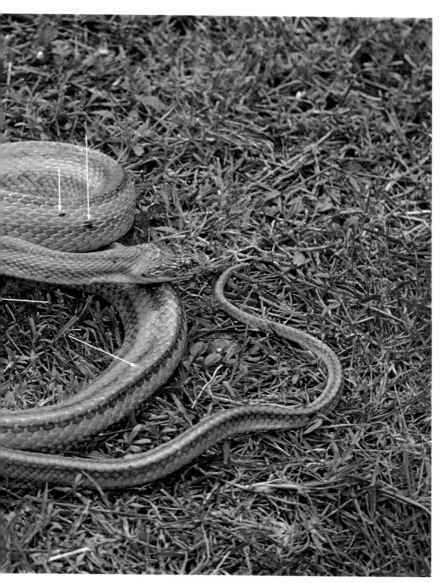

378. The rat snake *(Elaphe obsoleta)* shown in this picture had a small black patch in its skin which was removed by a veterinary surgeon; however, it was already too late. The tumor appeared in the form of numerous small black desposits disseminated over the snake's skin and gradually every part of the body was invaded. Photo: Grimstone.

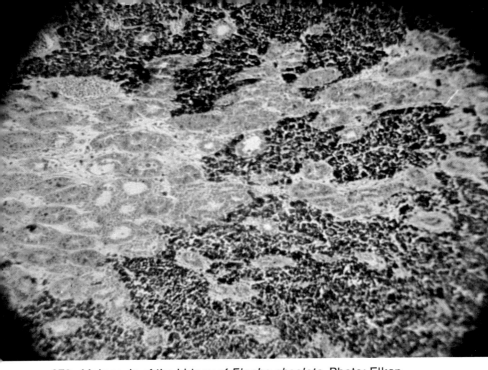

379. Melanosis of the kidney of *Elaphe obsoleta.* Photo: Elkan.

380. Melanosis of the fat body of *Elaphe obsoleta.* Photo: Elkan.

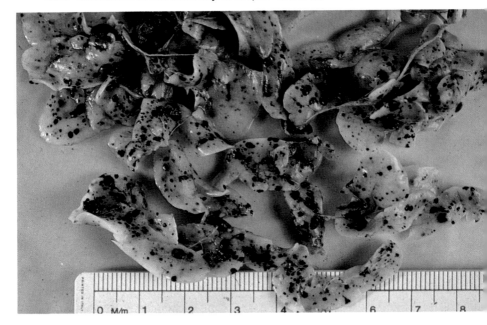

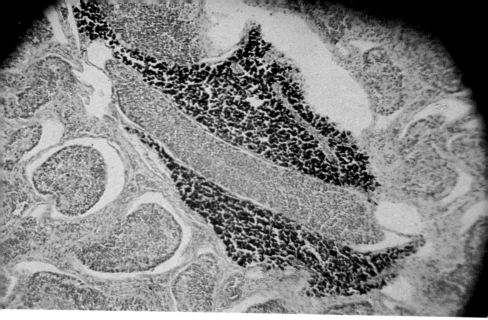

381. Melanotic deposit in the testis of *Elaphe obsoleta.* Photo: Elkan.

382. Melanotic deposit in the skin of *Elaphe obsoleta.* There is junctional activity at the junction of the dermis and epidermis. Photo: Elkan.

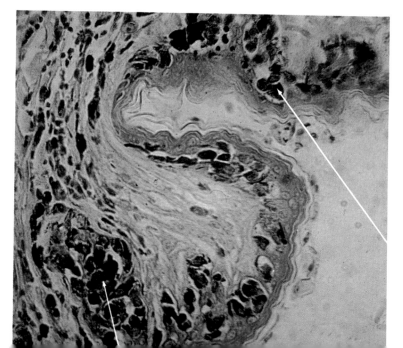

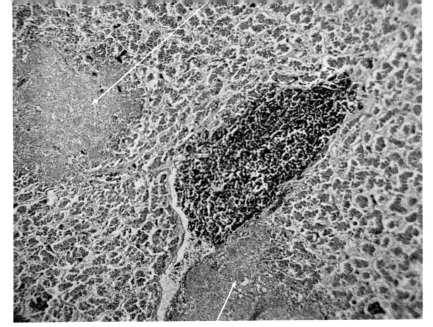

383. A melanotic deposit in the liver of *Elaphe obsoleta.* Two areas of necrosis due to *ante mortem* bacterial infection can be seen. Photo: Elkan.

384. Part of the melanotic tumor embedded in a thrombus found in the ventricle of the heart of *Elaphe obsoleta.* The tumor spreads by the blood stream. Photo: Elkan.

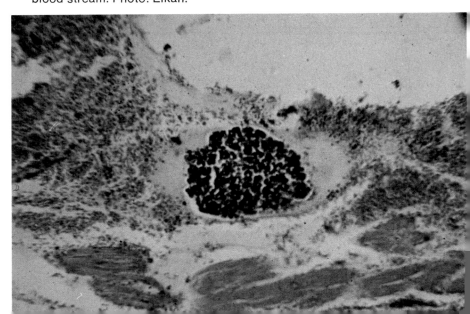

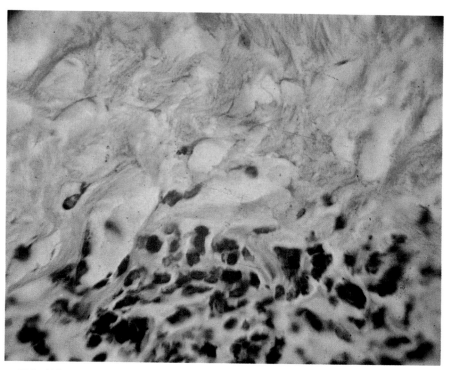

385. Where the melanotic tumor invades an area normally containing ground substance (upper half of picture), this substance (which consists mainly of mucopolysaccharides) disappears. It seems possible that the tumor feeds on the ground substance. Photo: Elkan.

HOST INDEX